DISC REPAIR BLUEPRINT

A Plan to Overcome Spinal Pain Through Cutting-Edge Technology and Old-School Wisdom. No Surgery Required.

By

DR. STEPHANIE A. MAJ

Dr. Stephanie A. Maj D.C.

Disc Repair Blueprint
Copyright © 2025 by Dr. Stephanie A. Maj
Perseverance Press Chicago, IL

ISBN: 979-8-218-59595-1

Contents

of Curis Functional Health-Chicago Lakeview

Social Media

Take the First Step Toward Better Health

Chapter 1
A Journey Through Pain and Radiculopathy: Why This Book Can Help

Have you ever paused and wondered why you're holding this book right now? It's no coincidence, I assure you. As a chiropractor dedicated to the art and science of movement, I've witnessed countless people bewildered by the forces that seem to conspire against them with age. Gravity, that unyielding force of nature, remains as constant as the earth's orbit. It pulls us down, while injuries seem to linger longer than they did in our youth. These ever-present forces shape our physical well-being in profound ways.

For much of our lives, we hold onto the false hope that time might somehow ease these burdens. The reality, however, is quite the opposite. As we age, gravity's impact intensifies, and injuries become more frequent. Our bodies grow more susceptible to the everyday strains and stresses. This book is your guide to understanding and navigating these natural, yet formidable, challenges. By turning these pages, you're stepping into a journey of confronting these realities and equipping yourself with the knowledge to flourish despite them.

Meet Dr. Stephanie Maj

Welcome to the transformative world of non-surgical spinal decompression—a groundbreaking approach in chiropractic care offering hope for those seeking relief from back pain without invasive procedures. My name is Dr. Stephanie Maj and as the Clinic Director of Curis Functional Health in Lakeview, Chicago, I am proud to lead this innovative practice. With over three decades of experience, my career has been dedicated to transforming lives through expertise in pediatric, pregnancy, and family wellness care.

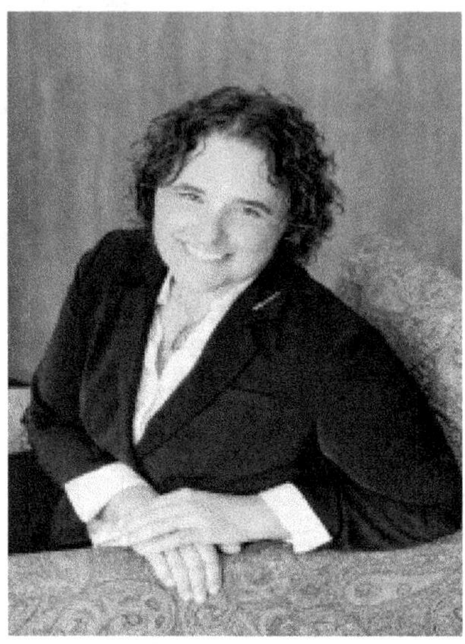

My approach to holistic health is comprehensive and rooted in my education—a Bachelor of Science in Clinical Nutrition and a Doctorate in Chiropractic. Certified in Pediatrics and the Webster Technique by the International Chiropractic Pediatric Association, my leadership extends beyond practice. I've served as president of the Royal Knights of the Chiropractic Roundtable and remain actively involved in The League of Chiropractic Women and the World Congress of Chiropractic Women.

As an author and podcast host, my book "You Can Be Well," and podcast "Women Seeking Wellness," have been platforms to share my insights. Through local initiatives, I've been privileged to support wellness within the unhoused communities in Chicago and abroad. I am asked to speak globally about a wide range of topics on health and vitality.

The Analogy that Explains it ALL

I feel compelled right now to tell you my pickle analogy. I

know that sounds very strange yet in my book, this was the most quoted, the most talked about and referenced story. It struck a cord with people and created an initiative to change.

How do you make a pickle? It's simple—you start with a fresh, crisp cucumber and immerse it in brine. Over time, the cucumber begins to transform. Now, here's an interesting thought—if you pull that cucumber out early enough in the process, it's still just a cucumber. You can rinse it off, dry it, and it's good as new. But once that cucumber has been in the brine too long, something irreversible happens. It crosses a line. It's no longer a cucumber—it's a pickle. At that point, no matter what you do, no matter how much effort you put in, you can't turn it back. It's a pickle forever.

Now, why does this story matter? Because your spine works in much the same way. When we're young, our spinal discs are like those fresh, vibrant cucumbers—hydrated, elastic, and resilient. These discs act as the cushions between your vertebrae, absorbing shock, supporting movement, and keeping your spine healthy and flexible. But just like the cucumber sitting in brine, over time, your spinal discs start to change. Everyday wear and tear, poor posture, injuries, or simply neglecting your spinal health can apply pressure to those discs. And as that pressure builds, the discs lose hydration, shrink, and deteriorate. Slowly but surely, the "brine" of life starts pulling the vitality out of them.

At some point, if left unchecked, those healthy discs cross a line. They lose their ability to recover, their capacity to cushion. They dry out, flatten, and degenerate to the point where the damage becomes permanent. This is the moment when your spine—like the cucumber—can no longer turn back. You've become… a pickle.

This transformation doesn't necessarily happen overnight. It takes years of accumulated stress and neglect, but by the time the pain sets in and mobility decreases, the pickle stage often feels unavoidable. And this is where so many people find themselves trudging down the difficult path of spinal pain, trying every last-ditch effort to turn back the clock, searching for some miracle fix. But as hard as it is to turn a pickle back into a cucumber, the goal is to stop before your spine decay gets to a point of no return (the pickle.)

This is where spinal decompression steps in like the hero to your spine's story. Imagine if you could catch that cucumber before it lingered too long in the brine. That's what spinal decompression does for your discs. It's a non-invasive treatment that gently stretches and elongates your spine, relieving the compressive pressures that have been squeezing the life—hydration and nutrients—out of your discs. With this release, your spine finally gets the chance to "breathe." Earth's natural forces, like gravity and daily wear, are temporarily eased, giving your discs the opportunity to absorb the nourishment they need to stay healthy.

Think of spinal decompression like pulling that cucumber out of the brine before it's too late. It's giving your spine a chance to rehydrate, heal, and recover, rather than continuing to deteriorate into a state of no return. This process doesn't just stop the damage in its tracks; it actively promotes regeneration by creating a nurturing environment for your spinal discs. They begin to plump back up, regaining their cushioning ability. Pressure on nerves is relieved, pain subsides, and mobility returns.

The thing about spinal decompression is that it works best when intervention happens early—when your spine is still in its cucumber stage. It's not just about repairing what's damaged; it's about preventing irreversible damage altogether. When you take care of your spine with therapies like decompression, you're effectively stopping that slow, brining process before it has the chance to take away the vibrancy of your spine's health.

But maybe you're reading this and thinking, "What if I've already started turning into a pickle? What if my spine has already crossed that line?" Here's the good news—the human body has incredible potential for healing, even if you feel like you're halfway into your pickle transformation. Spinal decompression can still help mitigate damage, improve mobility, and ease discomfort, even if it's harder to get back to that fresh cucumber state. The key is to take action now—because while you might not be able to undo everything, you can still make a huge difference in how your spine feels and functions moving forward.

Here's the truth we all need to hear—too many of us ignore the health of our spines. We start life as vibrant cucumbers, taking for granted our flexibility, our pain-free movement, and our resilience. We don't think much about the long-term consequences of poor posture, sedentary lifestyles, or skipping out on spinal care. Then one day, we wake up, and the changes are undeniable. We feel the stiffness, the pain, the limitations creeping in. That's why I wrote this book—because it doesn't have to get to that point.

Spinal decompression is your opportunity to reclaim your spine's health before it's too late. It's your chance to pull your cucumber out of the brine, to preserve its vitality, and to keep it functioning the way it's meant to. And if you're already feeling the strain? It's never too late to start. With the right care—whether it's decompression, chiropractic adjustments, or other therapies —you can slow the process, regain comfort, and keep moving forward with hope.

Your spine is worth the effort. Don't wait until it's too late. Act now. Take that first step toward spinal health and give your body the care it deserves, before the transformation becomes irreversible. Your cucumber deserves to thrive.

Chiropractic and Non-Surgical Spinal Decompression is at the Heart of It All

In this book, we delve into how non-surgical spinal

decompression, guided by professionals like myself, relieves pressure on spinal discs and promotes healing. This technique offers pain relief, increased mobility, and reduced nerve pressure while empowering the body's natural healing abilities. At Curis Functional Health, we invite you to embark on a recovery journey that respects your individual needs and promotes well-being, embodying the "Curis Way" by integrating chiropractic care with functional medicine and mental health support.

Integrating non-surgical spinal decompression enhances the care we offer, providing an alternative for chronic back pain sufferers who may not respond well to traditional adjustments or wish to avoid surgery. This approach allows us to address a broader range of spinal issues, tailoring treatment plans to diverse needs. Our commitment to holistic health solutions strengthens our reputation as a leader in comprehensive, cutting-edge care options, fostering trust and loyalty among our patients.

In my clinic, we serve as a sanctuary for every stage of health, guiding individuals from recovery to maintaining optimal wellness. My vision is to lead you toward health and wellness with compassion, expertise, and cutting-edge technology, placing chiropractic care as a cornerstone of your health journey.

Non-surgical spinal decompression stands out in chiropractic care as a sophisticated technique for alleviating back pain without invasive interventions. This approach is built on precision and gentle care, using advanced technology to address spinal discomfort's root causes.

At the heart of this technique is a motorized traction table, a tool enabling us to administer controlled, targeted decompression. By applying strategic traction forces, we carefully stretch the spine, relieving pressure on affected discs. This creates negative pressure, retracting herniated, arthritic, or bulging discs and alleviating nerve pressure.

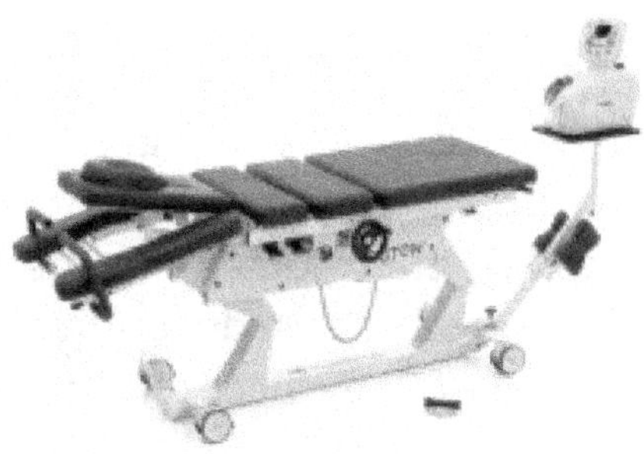

The benefits are multifaceted—significant pain relief, enhanced mobility, and reduced nerve pressure lead to renewed well-being. This method not only provides immediate relief but fosters long-term spinal health, promoting proper alignment and hydration crucial for vertebral integrity.

Integrating non-surgical spinal decompression into holistic chiropractic care represents our commitment to comprehensive patient treatment. It complements manual adjustments, nutritional guidance, and lifestyle advice, creating a well-rounded strategy for spinal health and overall wellness. With personalized and cutting-edge care, we ensure your unique needs are addressed with expertise and empathy.

Reflecting on non-surgical spinal decompression, it's clear this approach offers immediate relief and long-term health benefits. It empowers individuals to reclaim vitality and enjoy life without chronic pain. Consider this transformative treatment option and engage with qualified chiropractors to guide you through spinal health. By exploring non-surgical spinal decompression, you embark on a path toward sustainable wellness and a more active life.

The Hidden Heroes of Healing

But here's where the magic of healing truly comes together. Spinal decompression creates the space, while chiropractic care ensures alignment and balance. And then, there are glycosaminoglycans—those tiny, powerful molecules you've probably never thought about but are vital for your spinal health.

Glycosaminoglycans (or GAGs) are like the "hydration specialists" of your discs. They're what help your discs retain water, stay elastic, and do their job as the cushions between your vertebrae. When there's injury or degeneration, your discs lose these essential molecules. They become dried out, stiff, and far more prone to damage.

But the incredible thing is that GAG levels can be replenished. With the right nutrients, targeted therapies, and consistent care, your body can begin to rebuild these vital building blocks. It's a bit like planting seeds in a garden—at first, the changes aren't visible, but with time, nourishment, and effort, growth happens.

When GAGs are restored, your spinal discs regain their flexibility, their bounce, and their ability to support you without pain or resistance. This isn't just about avoiding more damage; it's about genuinely restoring what was lost.

The Mind-Body Connection in Chronic Pain

Living with chronic pain isn't just about physical discomfort —it impacts every aspect of life, from emotional well-being to daily interactions. The constant struggle with pain can lead to frustration, anxiety, and even depression, creating a cycle where emotional distress worsens the physical experience. Tasks that once felt effortless become daunting, social connections fade due to withdrawal, and the sense of control over one's health diminishes. The mind and body are deeply connected, and without addressing both, true healing remains out of reach.

At Curis Functional Health, we recognize that pain relief requires more than just physical treatment—it demands a whole-person approach. That's why we integrate cutting-edge therapies like non-surgical spinal decompression with functional medicine and mental health support. Counseling, including evidence-based techniques like cognitive behavioral therapy and mindfulness, helps patients break free from the emotional weight of chronic pain. By treating both the body and mind, we empower patients to regain strength, confidence, and control over their health—because true healing goes beyond symptom relief.

My Hope for You Is a Life Free from Drugs and Surgery

When I decided to write this book, it wasn't just about sharing knowledge; it was about saving lives—maybe even your life. I've seen too many people fall into the heartbreaking cycle of failed back syndrome and opiate addiction, and it's something I just couldn't sit back and ignore. It usually starts with good intentions—someone seeks relief from unrelenting back pain and is told surgery is the only option. But when that first surgery doesn't work, another is recommended, and sometimes another after that. Each procedure takes a toll, both physically and emotionally, leaving people with even more pain, less hope, and no clear way forward. And then there's the prescription for painkillers—a quick fix that can snowball into dependency before you even realize what's happening. What starts as an attempt to "feel better" turns into an overwhelming burden of chronic pain and addiction that's nearly impossible to escape.

You Can Be Well!

But here's the thing—it doesn't have to get to that point. That's why this book exists. Writing it wasn't just about highlighting the challenges people face, but about showing you that there's a better way. It's about offering solutions like spinal decompression and other non-surgical treatments that can help relieve pain and restore function without the risks that come with invasive procedures or addictive medications. Spinal decompression, for example, gives your spine the chance to heal naturally, addressing the root cause of the issue rather than masking symptoms or creating new problems. It's an option that far too many people don't even know exists, and I couldn't stand by knowing that information like this—life-changing, empowering information—wasn't reaching the people who need it most.

I've seen the relief in a person's eyes when they've finally found a solution that works after years of suffering. I've talked to people who had all but given up, who thought they'd spend their lives trapped in endless pain or relying on pills to just get through the day. Seeing that kind of transformation—helping someone regain hope, mobility, and freedom—is exactly why I'm so passionate about this work. I want you to know that you have choices—choices that don't involve handing over your future to risky surgeries or suffocating under the weight of addiction.

This book is a guide, but it's also a conversation between us. I wrote it because I know the frustration, the fear, and the exhaustion that can come with chronic pain. But I also know there's hope. And I want you to feel that. You can take control of your spinal health, explore alternative treatments, and step off the path that's led so many others to heartbreak. You deserve better —you deserve to know that there is a way forward, that your life doesn't have to revolve around pain or the fear of it. Writing this book was my way of reaching out to you, of saying, "You're not alone in this, and there's a way out." Your healing starts with the knowledge and choices you make today, and I'm here to help you find a path that changes everything for the better.

Chapter 2
Anatomy of the Spine and Disc Injuries

To really understand non-surgical spinal decompression, it helps to know a bit about how the spine works and how injuries happen. This chapter breaks down the structure and function of the spine, along with common disc injuries like herniation, bulging, and degeneration. The more you know about your body, the easier it is to see how spinal decompression can make a difference.

Anatomy of the Spine

The spine, a marvel of human anatomy, is made up of 33 vertebrae organized into five regions, each with unique characteristics and purposes. At the top, the cervical spine includes seven vertebrae (C1–C7) responsible for supporting the head's weight and providing exceptional mobility for gestures like nodding and turning the head. C1, the atlas, and C2, the axis, are distinct in their design, facilitating the head's rotational movement. Beneath this lies the thoracic spine, comprising of 12 vertebrae (T1–T12) that provide stability and serve as attachment points for ribs, forming a protective cage around vital organs like the heart and lungs. Moving downward, the lumbar region features five strong vertebrae (L1–L5), engineered to carry the majority of the body's weight and permit movements such as bending forward and lifting objects. Following this, the sacrum consists of five fused vertebrae that connect the spine to the pelvis, forming a sturdy base for the upper body. Lastly, the coccygeal spine, or tailbone, consists of four fused vertebrae that provide structural support to the pelvic area and serve as attachment sites for tendons and muscles.

Each vertebra is intricately designed to balance strength and mobility. The vertebral body, a thick cylindrical structure, handles weight-bearing responsibilities and is composed of a spongy interior encased in a strong exterior shell for shock absorption. Extending behind the body, the vertebral arch surrounds the vertebral foramen, a hollow space that houses and protects the delicate spinal cord. Protruding from the arch are various processes—such as the spinous and transverse processes—serving as connection points for muscles and ligaments that stabilize and mobilize the spine. The aligned openings between adjacent vertebrae, called intervertebral foramina, allow spinal nerves to exit the spinal cord and branch out through the body, controlling movement and transmitting sensory information.

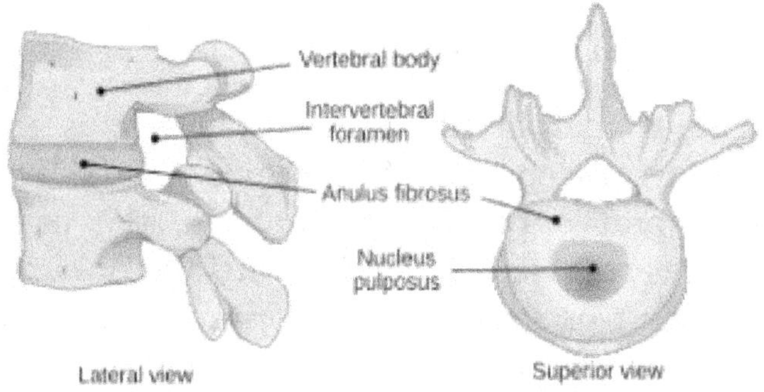

Intervertebral discs, positioned between most vertebrae, are essential for both spinal flexibility and endurance. These discs act like cushions, absorbing stress and allowing the spine to bend, twist, and stretch. Their structure can be likened to an onion, with layers of increasing complexity that work together to maintain their essential function. The outermost "layers" of the disc—called the annulus fibrosus—are tight, concentric rings of collagen fibers. Much like the tough, fibrous outer layers of an onion protect it from damage, the annulus fibrosus resists tearing and provides sturdy containment for the inner material. Deeper into the disc, past these fibrous layers, lies the "core" or "heart" of the onion—the nucleus pulposus. This gelatinous central portion is rich in water and proteins, allowing it to deform under pressure and rebound to its original shape when the load is removed. This enables the nucleus pulposus to distribute pressure evenly across the disc and vertebral bodies, much like the soft core of an onion ensures structural integrity through its ability to compress and return to form.

Together, the vertebrae and intervertebral discs form a synergistic system that protects the spine, supports body weight, and allows fluid motion. The vertebrae shield the spinal cord, while their processes and arrangement enable control over posture and movement. The onion-like intervertebral discs amplify this protection and flexibility by absorbing shocks from actions like walking, running, or lifting. As we bend, twist, or extend, the discs adapt by redistributing force across their complex layers, preventing damage or excessive wear to the vertebrae. This integrated design ensures that the spine can withstand daily stresses while maintaining spinal cord integrity and enabling the extensive range of motion required for human activity.

Areas Vulnerable to Injury and Decay

The cervical and lumbar regions of the spine are particularly prone to disc injuries due to a combination of anatomical, functional, and mechanical factors that subject these areas to increased stress over time. Starting with the cervical spine, this part of the spine consists of seven small vertebrae (C1 to C7) located in the neck and is built for flexibility rather than stability. Its primary role is to support the weight of the head—approximately 10 to 15 pounds—and to facilitate an impressive range of motion, including nodding, rotation, and side-to-side tilting. However, this high degree of mobility comes at the cost of vulnerability. The cervical intervertebral discs, which cushion and allow smooth movements between these vertebrae, are under constant dynamic pressure—quick turns, sudden jerks, or prolonged awkward head positions (like looking down at a screen) can lead to strain or microdamage in the disc structure. Over time, these stresses can weaken the annulus fibrosus, the tough outer layer of the disc, allowing the softer nucleus pulposus inside to bulge or even herniate, pressing against nearby spinal nerves. Common activities like driving, desk work, texting or even sleeping in a poor position can exacerbate this risk.

The lumbar spine, located in the lower back, is likewise prone to injury, albeit for slightly different reasons. This region consists of five large, weight-bearing vertebrae (L1 to L5) that support most of the body's weight above the pelvis while also acting as a critical point of flexibility for movements like bending, twisting, and lifting. Unlike the cervical spine, the lumbar spine is not designed for extreme flexibility but rather for a balance of movement and strength. However, due to its role in bearing heavy loads and frequent mechanical stress, the lumbar intervertebral discs are particularly susceptible to wear and tear over time. Everyday activities like bending to pick up objects, twisting while carrying heavy loads, or even prolonged periods of sitting can place relentless compressive and shear forces on the lumbar discs. These movements make the lumbar discs work harder to absorb the impacts, increasing the likelihood of annular tears or nucleus pulposus herniation.

Another critical factor contributing to the vulnerability of both the cervical and lumbar spine is the limited external support they receive compared to the thoracic spine. The thoracic spine is protected and stabilized by the ribcage, which distributes forces more evenly and limits extreme motion. By contrast, the cervical and lumbar regions lack such reinforcement, leaving them exposed to a combination of mechanical and postural stresses. Poor posture—whether it's slouching in a chair, standing unevenly, or holding the head in a forward-leaning position—is another significant contributor to disc injuries. For example, prolonged forward head posture, often referred to as "tech neck," places increased strain on the cervical spine, compressing the discs and accelerating degeneration. Similarly, poor lower back posture during sitting or lifting can increase pressure on the lumbar discs, making them more prone to injury.

Age-related degeneration is another important factor that heightens the vulnerability of these regions. Over the years, the intervertebral discs naturally lose hydration and elasticity, a process that reduces their ability to absorb shocks and return to their original shape. This degeneration often begins in the lumbar discs, as they endure the highest loads, but can also develop in the cervical spine due to repetitive stresses and micro-traumas accumulated over time. Degenerated discs are more likely to bulge or herniate, especially when subjected to additional strain from sudden movements, heavy lifting, or high-impact activities.

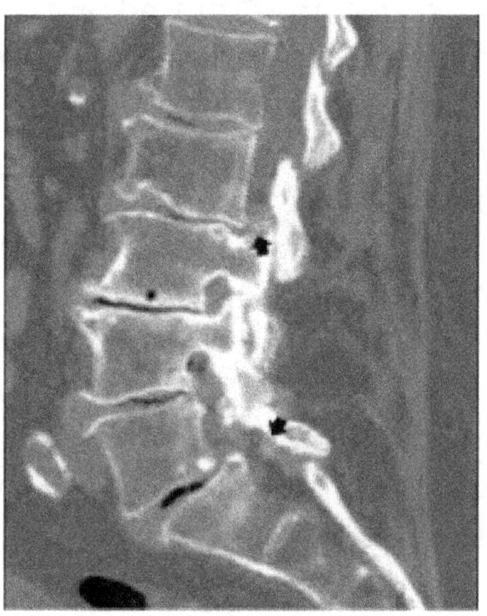

Repetitive stress is a compounding issue for individuals whose daily routines involve sustained or repeated motions that target these spinal regions. Athletes, for instance, who engage in activities requiring repeated neck movements (like in martial arts or gymnastics) or frequent bending and twisting of the lower back (as seen in weightlifting or golf) are at particularly high risk. Even everyday habits, like carrying heavy bags on one shoulder or sleeping on an unsupportive mattress, can place consistent, uneven stress on specific discs, accelerating the risk of injury.

The combination of high mobility, heavy mechanical demands, poor reinforcement, postural habits, repetitive stress, and age-related degeneration makes the cervical and lumbar spine the most common locations for disc injuries. Their integral role in both movement and weight-bearing means they are constantly tasked with balancing flexibility and stability, rendering these regions uniquely vulnerable to wear, strain, and damage over the course of a lifetime.

Neuropathy: How Pain in Arms, Hands, Legs, and Feet Can Come from the Spine

When a spinal disc becomes injured or arthritic, it can lead to nerve compression and associated neuropathies, with profound effects in both the cervical (neck) and lumbar (low back) regions. Neuropathy is a condition that happens when nerves in your body are damaged or not working properly. Nerves act like messengers, sending signals about sensations like touch, pain, or temperature to your brain and also control how your muscles move. When they're damaged, you might feel things like tingling, numbness, burning pain, or even weakness, often in areas like your hands or feet. Neuropathy can have many causes, including diabetes, injuries, or infections. Our focus is on problems like a herniated disc that puts pressure on nearby nerves. It's your body's way of telling you something's wrong with these important communication pathways, and pinpointing the cause is key to finding the right treatment.

Spinal discs act as essential shock absorbers between vertebrae, but when they deteriorate due to injury, wear, or arthritis, they can protrude or herniate into the space occupied by nerve roots or even larger nerve plexuses. This compression disrupts signaling pathways, causing pain, numbness, weakness, and other sensory or motor impairments.

Cervical Spine and the Brachial Plexus:

Disc injuries in the neck most commonly affect the cervical spine, where nerve roots belong to or contribute to the brachial plexus. This network of nerves extends from the spinal cord through the lower neck and shoulder areas, giving rise to the nerves that control sensation and movement in the shoulders, arms, and hands. When cervical discs deteriorate or herniate, they can irritate or compress nerve roots, leading to conditions like cervical radiculopathy. For example, a herniated disc at the C5-C6 level might compress the sixth cervical nerve root, resulting in symptoms such as pain radiating into the arm, weakness in the biceps, difficulty extending the wrist, and altered sensations in the thumb or index finger. Since the brachial plexus is so integral to upper limb function, injuries or degenerative changes in the cervical spine can severely impact mobility and dexterity, hindering daily activities like lifting, gripping, or writing.

Lumbar Spine, Sciatic Nerve, and the Sacral Plexus:

The lower back, home to the lumbar spine, often bears the brunt of disc-related neuropathies because of the immense physical stress and weight it endures. Disc injuries at the L4-L5 or L5-S1 levels are particularly problematic, as they frequently compress the nerve roots that contribute to the sacral plexus. This plexus is a critical nerve network that gives rise to the sciatic nerve—the largest nerve in the body. The sciatic nerve runs from the lower back, through the buttocks, and down both legs, supplying sensation and motor control to much of the lower body. Herniation or arthritis in the lumbar discs can irritate or pinch these nerve roots, leading to sciatica.

Understanding Sciatica:

Sciatica is a specific type of neuropathy characterized by sharp, often debilitating pain radiating from the lower back, through the buttock, and down the back or side of the leg, potentially reaching the foot. Depending on the location and severity of the disc compression, additional symptoms may include tingling, numbness, muscle weakness, and difficulty controlling or moving the leg or foot. For example, compression of the L4-L5 nerve root could cause weakness in extending the big toe, while L5-S1 compression may result in difficulty standing on the toes and sensory loss along the outer foot. These symptoms may worsen with movements like bending, sitting for extended periods, or lifting, which increase pressure on the lumbar region.

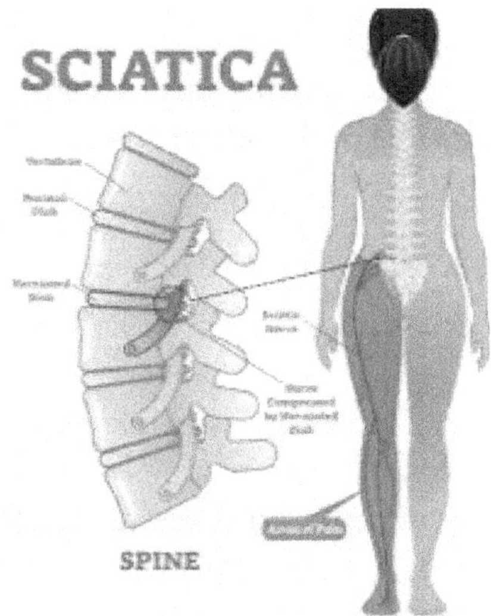

The impact of sciatica extends beyond physical discomfort. It can significantly impair walking, sitting, and performing routine tasks. Chronic cases may result in muscle atrophy or permanent nerve damage if untreated. Spinal decompression therapy is a common non-invasive treatment for sciatica, designed to alleviate nerve compression by creating space between vertebrae and promoting disc retraction and healing.

Understanding how the brachial and sacral plexuses function within these regions provides additional insight into the complexity and interconnectedness of disc-related neuropathies. The nerves they house are finely tuned systems responsible for relaying critical signals between the spine and limbs. When displaced or irritated by an injured or arthritic disc, the resulting symptoms remind us how vital these networks are to movement and sensation. Early treatment, including therapies like spinal decompression, chiropractic, or targeted exercises, can often restore comfort and mobility, empowering individuals to regain control over their health and quality of life.

Chapter 3
Introduction to Spinal Decompression

Non-surgical spinal decompression is an innovative and non-invasive therapy designed to relieve pressure on the spine and alleviate chronic back pain. This treatment works by gently stretching the spine using advanced equipment such as the Chattanooga Triton Decompression Unit, a state-of-the-art machine specifically engineered for precision and comfort. By creating negative pressure within the spinal discs, this process encourages herniated, bulging, or arthritic discs to retract, promoting natural healing and improving the flow of oxygen, water, and nutrient-rich fluids into the discs. It's a safe, effective option for individuals looking to manage back pain without surgery or medication, offering a path to long-term relief and improved mobility.

In this chapter, we'll go over the fundamentals of spinal decompression, how it works and differs from other forms of treatment. You'll gain a basic understanding of what happens to your spine during therapy and the potential benefits you can experience.

Just a little history...

Non-surgical spinal decompression has a fascinating and progressive history, rooted in humanity's ongoing effort to develop safe, non-invasive treatments for spinal conditions. The therapy evolved from traditional spinal traction methods, which date back centuries and were used to alleviate back and joint pain through mechanical stretching. While early traction systems provided some relief, they lacked precision and adaptability, often proving ineffective for severe disc-related conditions. Spurred by a deeper understanding of spinal biomechanics in the mid-20th century, researchers began exploring more targeted techniques designed explicitly to address intervertebral disc problems.

One of the pivotal figures in this evolution was Dr. Allan Dyer, a Canadian physician, biomedical engineer, and former Deputy Minister of Health for Ontario. Dr. Dyer is widely credited with pioneering computerized spinal decompression technology. He recognized the limitations of conventional traction and sought to develop a method that could apply precise, controlled forces to the spine, targeting specific disc issues without causing additional strain or discomfort. His early innovations laid the groundwork for non-surgical spinal decompression, combining mechanical principles with advanced technology to offer a more effective solution for conditions like herniated discs, sciatica, neuropathy and degenerative disc disease.

Non-surgical spinal decompression has been in use for several decades, evolving from traditional traction therapies. The technique gained prominence in the late 20th century, particularly with the development of computerized systems like the Chattanooga Triton Decompression Unit. The underlying science behind spinal decompression is both intricate and elegant. During treatment, this specialized unit gently stretches the spine in a controlled and progressive manner. This creates negative pressure—or intradiscal decompression—within the intervertebral discs. Negative pressure works in two key ways. First, it encourages herniated or bulging disc material to retract back into the disc's center, relieving the pressure on surrounding nerves that is often the source of pain and discomfort. Second, it stimulates improved blood flow and nutrient exchange within the disc. These nutrients are critical for repairing damaged disc tissues, promoting natural healing, and reducing inflammation. Unlike traditional traction, which applies a uniform pull, spinal decompression uses advanced algorithms to cycle between gentle pulling and relaxation phases. This dynamic adjustment prevents the musculature from resisting the stretch, allowing for deeper and more effective decompression.

Modern technology has vastly enhanced the precision and customization of non-surgical spinal decompression. Machines like the Chattanooga Triton Decompression Unit are equipped with advanced software to adjust treatment protocols, tailoring them to each patient's unique spinal anatomy and condition. These devices can focus on specific areas of the spine, whether it's the cervical (neck) or lumbar (lower back) regions, and adapt to the severity of the disc injury. Additionally, the equipment includes safety features that ensure the stretch remains within a comfortable and therapeutic range, enhancing both the effectiveness and the patient experience.

Chiropractic Care and Non-surgical Spinal Decompression

The development of non-surgical spinal decompression represents a significant leap forward in spinal care. It bridges the gap between traditional chiropractic methods, which often rely on manual adjustments, and invasive surgical procedures that carry risks and extended recovery times. By offering a non-invasive, drug-free, and highly targeted approach, spinal decompression has become a go-to therapy for individuals seeking relief from debilitating back pain, sciatica, and other disc-related conditions. Its ability to address the root causes of these issues, rather than just masking symptoms, has made it a mainstay in modern chiropractic practice.

When it comes to addressing back pain, sciatica, or disc-related problems, non-surgical spinal decompression and regular chiropractic care are two effective, non-invasive options, each offering unique benefits. Non-surgical spinal decompression stands out as a specialized therapy for conditions like herniated discs, bulging discs, sciatica, and degenerative disc disease.

Using advanced equipment such as the Chattanooga Triton Decompression Unit, this method gently stretches the spine in a controlled manner, creating negative pressure. This process allows herniated or bulging discs to retract, easing pressure on nerves and reducing inflammation. Additionally, it encourages nutrient-rich blood flow to the damaged areas, promoting natural healing. Best of all, this approach is entirely non-invasive and drug-free, offering a safe alternative to surgery with no downtime. The therapy can also be customized to fit each patient's specific condition, making it an adaptable and highly targeted treatment option.

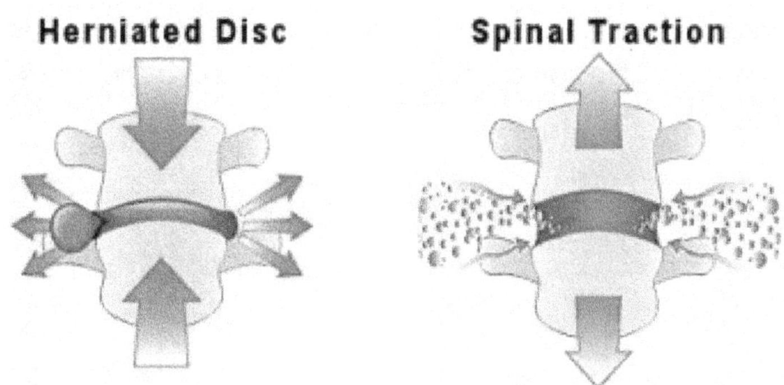

On the other hand, regular chiropractic care focuses on improving spinal alignment and overall function through manual adjustments. Chiropractors use their hands or specialized tools to reposition misaligned vertebrae, which can enhance nerve function, encouraging healing and relief of pain. While spinal decompression targets disc-specific issues, chiropractic care takes a broader approach, addressing various musculoskeletal and nervous system concerns, including general back pain, stiffness, posture-related issues, and even headaches. This method also prioritizes whole-body wellness by ensuring proper spinal alignment and supporting the body's natural healing processes.

The key differences between these treatments lie in their focus and techniques. Non-surgical spinal decompression directly treats disc-related conditions by applying negative pressure to the spine, facilitating disc retraction and healing. Meanwhile, chiropractic adjustments work to restore alignment and mobility, addressing discomfort caused by vertebral subluxations.

Choosing between these therapies depends on your specific needs. For disc-related problems like herniation or sciatica, decompression therapy offers precision and long-lasting relief. For general alignment issues or a more holistic approach to spinal health, chiropractic adjustments are highly effective. Many practitioners combine both methods to maximize outcomes, pairing the targeted nature of spinal decompression with the broader benefits of chiropractic care. Whichever path you choose, both approaches empower you to take control of your health, offering non-invasive routes to pain relief, improved mobility, and better overall well-being.

Chapter 4
Common Disc Injuries: Understanding Herniated Discs, Bulging Discs, and Degenerative Disc Disease

T he human spine is pretty amazing—it keeps us stable, lets us move, bend, and tackle daily life with ease. A big part of what makes this possible are the intervertebral discs, those soft, cushiony pads between the vertebrae. They act like shock absorbers, support the spine, and help us move smoothly. But, like any hardworking part of the body, these discs can run into trouble. Issues like herniated discs, bulging discs, and degenerative disc disease (DDD) are very common and can cause discomfort or even pain. Each condition affects the spine differently, with its own set of causes, symptoms, and treatments.

Herniated Discs

A herniated disc is a condition where the inner gel-like core of a disc, called the nucleus pulposus, pushes through a tear or weakness in the tough outer layer known as the annulus fibrosus. This condition typically results from excessive pressure or tear-and-wear caused by repetitive stress over time. It is most commonly seen in the cervical (neck) and lumbar (lower back) regions of the spine, where mobility and mechanical stress are greatest. Causes for herniated discs may include improper lifting techniques, sudden twisting motions, traumatic injuries (such as car accidents), or any activity that places intense strain on the spine. Additionally, age-related degeneration makes the annulus fibrosus weaker and more likely to rupture, especially when coupled with repetitive day-to-day activities. The symptoms of a herniated disc vary depending on its location and the degree of nerve compression. If the herniation compresses a nearby nerve, it may result in radicular pain—sharp, shooting pain that radiates along the length of the affected nerve. For example, a herniated disc in the lumbar spine may cause sciatica, characterized by pain radiating from the lower back down one leg. Other symptoms may include tingling, numbness, muscle weakness, or, in severe cases, issues with bowel or bladder control, which could indicate a medical emergency. Treatment options for herniated discs range from noninvasive to surgical. Conservative methods often include chiropractic to restore alignment, calm nerves, improve flexibility and strength, anti-inflammatory diet and supplements to reduce swelling. Of course, non-surgical spinal decompression can help draw the herniation back to the center of the disc.

As an absolute last resort, surgical interventions like microdiscectomy may be necessary to remove the herniated portion of the disc and relieve nerve compression. The problem is that Failed Back Surgery Syndrome (FBSS) is a condition that occurs when a patient experiences persistent pain in their back or legs after undergoing spine surgery. Up to 40% of back surgeries result in FBSS, so surgery is the last resort intervention.

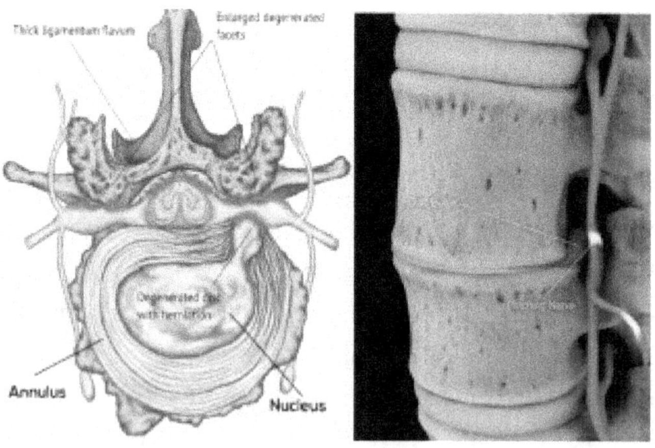

Bulging Discs

A bulging disc is considered a milder form of disc injury. Unlike a herniated disc, where the inner material escapes, a bulging disc involves a deformation of the disc as the nucleus pulposus shifts, causing the outer layer to bulge outward but remain intact. While not always symptomatic, a bulging disc can still exert pressure on nearby nerves or the spinal cord, leading to discomfort and other issues. Causes of bulging discs often parallel those of herniated discs, including poor posture, repetitive spinal strain, obesity, and age-related wear. Prolonged sedentary behavior and physically demanding occupations are also significant contributors. Bulging discs are commonly found in the lumbar and cervical spine, as these regions handle the majority of the body's movement and weight-bearing functions. The symptoms of bulging discs can range from mild stiffness or localized pain to more pronounced nerve-related symptoms, such as radiating pain, numbness, or a pins-and-needles sensation. However, many bulging discs remain asymptomatic until further degeneration occurs or a triggering event increases inflammation and nerve compression.

Degenerative Disc Disease (DDD)

Degenerative Disc Disease is a natural, age-related condition that affects the structure and function of the intervertebral discs. Despite its name, it is not a disease but rather a progressive breakdown caused by the gradual loss of water content and elasticity in the discs. Over time, this degeneration reduces the discs' ability to absorb shocks, making the spine more vulnerable to injuries such as herniation or bulging. The causes of DDD stem primarily from aging, but lifestyle factors like a sedentary routine, smoking, repetitive heavy lifting, and poor posture can accelerate the process. Genetics also play a role; some individuals are predisposed to faster disc degeneration. Symptoms of DDD vary widely. Early signs may include chronic back or neck pain, especially during movement or after prolonged periods of sitting or standing. Limited mobility, stiffness, and occasional shooting pain in the limbs are also common. As the condition progresses, nerve compression may lead to radiating symptoms or muscle weakness. While DDD cannot be reversed, treatment focuses on symptom relief and preserving function.

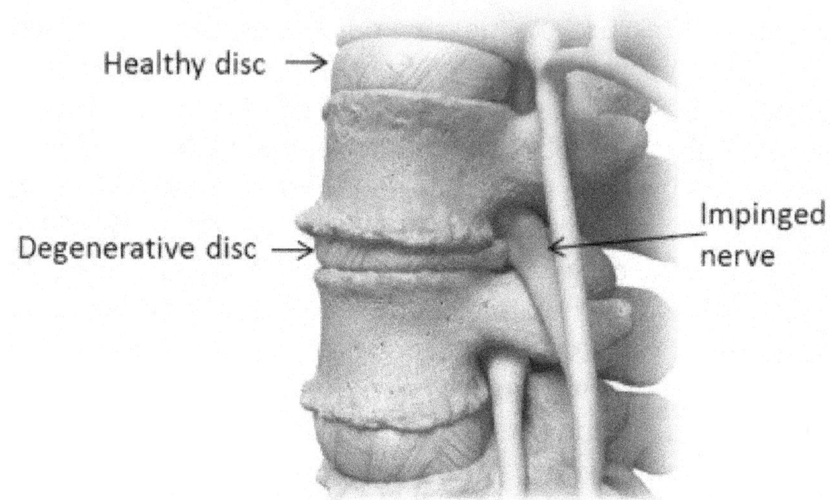

Nerve Compression and Its Implications

A common consequence of all three conditions is nerve compression, which can severely impact mobility and quality of life. Compressed nerves cause pain, tingling, numbness, and weakness along the affected nerve's pathway. For instance, compression in the cervical spine can affect the shoulders, arms, and hands, while nerve issues in the lumbar spine often impact the lower body. Prolonged compression can lead to more severe complications, making early intervention critical.

Lifestyle Factors and Prevention

Certain lifestyle factors significantly influence the development and progression of disc injuries. Obesity increases the mechanical load on the spine, accelerating disc wear. Poor posture, particularly during prolonged sitting or repetitive activities, misaligns the spine and increases strain. Sedentary habits weaken the muscles surrounding the spine, reducing its ability to absorb impacts efficiently. To reduce the risk of disc injuries, adopting preventive measures is crucial. Regular exercise focusing on flexibility and core strength can stabilize the spine. Low-impact activities such as swimming, gentle yoga, or walking can improve circulation and support discs. Proper lifting techniques—bending at the knees instead of the waist—can minimize strain on the lower back. Maintaining a healthy weight and avoiding smoking are additional steps to enhance disc longevity.

How Non-Surgical Spinal Decompression can Address Common Disc Injuries

Spinal injuries such as herniated discs, bulging discs, and degenerative disc disease can significantly impact a person's quality of life. The resulting symptoms—back and neck pain, nerve compression, weakness, and reduced mobility—often create a cycle of discomfort and physical limitations. Non-surgical spinal decompression offers a promising treatment alternative tailored to address these common disc injuries without the need for invasive procedures. By relieving pressure, enhancing healing, and restoring function, this technique has become an appealing option for individuals seeking long-term relief.

Benefits and Outcomes of Spinal Decompression

One of the significant benefits of non-surgical spinal decompression is its non-invasive nature. The treatment avoids the risks often associated with surgical interventions, such as infection, long recovery times, or complications from anesthesia. It does not require incisions, making it a low-risk option for those hesitant or unable to pursue surgery.

Patients undergoing non-surgical spinal decompression

typically experience a reduction in pain levels, improved mobility, and enhanced physical function over a series of treatment sessions. It is particularly effective for managing chronic pain associated with nerve root compression. For instance, individuals who suffer from sciatica—a condition where the sciatic nerve is compressed, often due to a lumbar disc injury—often report relief in leg and lower back pain after spinal decompression treatments.

The therapy is gentle, with treatments typically lasting about 15 minutes per session. A personalized treatment plan is developed based on the specific type and severity of the disc injury, ensuring that the procedure targets the affected spinal area effectively. This adaptability makes it suitable for a broad range of spinal conditions, from minor disc bulges to advanced degenerative issues.

Additionally, spinal decompression can often serve as a complementary treatment to physical therapy, providing a foundation of pain relief and increased mobility that allows patients to engage more fully in exercises designed to strengthen and stabilize the spine. This dual approach aids in long-term success by addressing both immediate symptoms and the underlying causes of disc injuries.

A Hopeful Path to Healing

Non-surgical spinal decompression offers hope for those grappling with the life-altering effects of common disc injuries. By relieving pressure, reducing nerve irritation, and stimulating the body's natural mechanisms for repair, this therapy helps break the cycle of chronic pain and debilitation. For individuals who have struggled to find relief through other methods, spinal decompression serves as a beacon of possibility—enabling them to regain mobility, reduce pain, and return to an active and empowered life.

If you've felt held back by herniated discs, bulging discs,

or degenerative disc disease, exploring non-surgical spinal decompression with your healthcare provider could be the first step toward reclaiming control over your spinal health and achieving the quality of life you deserve. The road to healing may take time, but with the right treatment and a proactive mindset, brighter days—free of pain—are well within reach.

Chapter 5
Revolutionizing Spinal Care: The Chattanooga Triton Decompression Unit

The Triton is one of the few decompression units that uses advanced traction algorithms designed to mimic the natural movements of the spine. These cutting-edge algorithms adapt dynamically to each patient's needs, offering a personalized and effective treatment experience. By constantly responding to small changes in the patient's condition during therapy, the Triton ensures targeted pressure is applied where it's needed most, resulting in optimal decompression. This smart, adaptive approach not only boosts the therapeutic effects but also reduces the risk of muscle guarding—a common issue with older, static systems. Muscle guarding, where muscles tighten to protect themselves, can slow recovery and prolong discomfort, making the Triton's technology a real game-changer. Studies show that adaptive systems like the Triton help speed up recovery, improve spinal alignment, and provide longer-lasting pain relief compared to traditional methods. Simply put, the Triton doesn't just treat spinal issues more effectively—it also supports long-term healing and better functionality, setting a new standard in non-surgical care.

Getting Comfortable on the Triton Unit

When it's time for your session on the Triton unit, the process is simple, smooth, and designed with your comfort in mind. This advanced device is used to help improve your spinal health and provide much-needed relief, and our staff is here to guide you every step of the way. Here's what you can expect when you're placed on the Triton unit:

First, we'll start by getting you settled into the treatment room. It's a quiet, calming space that's meant to make you feel relaxed from the get-go. The Triton unit itself is an impressive device, with a sleek, modern design and cushioned surfaces to keep you comfortable throughout your session. Don't worry if it looks a little technical—that just means it's packed with features that will tailor your treatment to your unique needs.

Next, one of our friendly team members will walk you through the process, answering any questions you might have. We'll take a moment to talk about how you've been feeling and the goals for this session, whether it's relieving pressure, improving alignment, or addressing pinched nerves. This conversation ensures your treatment is customized to suit your specific condition.

Once you're ready, we'll help you lie down on the Triton unit. Positioning is key here, and we'll work carefully to make sure you're in just the right spot. You'll start by lying flat on your back or stomach, depending on the type of treatment we're doing. Don't worry—we'll explain why one position might be better for you than the other. The table is fully padded and designed to support your body gently but firmly, so there are no pressure points or awkward spots.

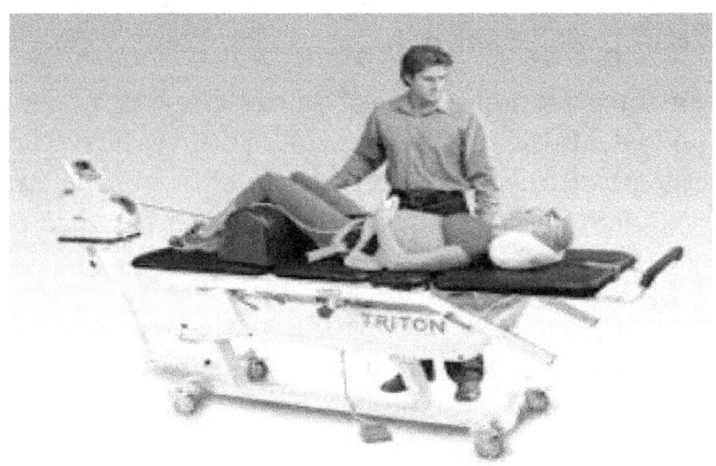

At this stage, we'll secure you on the table with comfortable straps or harnesses. This ensures that you stay in the optimal position during the treatment and allows the Triton to do its job effectively. For instance, if we're targeting your lower back, the harness might help isolate that specific area while keeping the rest of your body stable. Rest assured, these straps are snug yet soft— they're designed to keep you secure without any discomfort.

The Triton unit also has adjustable sections so we can align the table perfectly with your body's natural form. This feature is one of the things patients love most, as it prevents any added strain and keeps the experience as relaxing as possible.

Before the treatment begins, we'll double-check everything— your position, the strap placement, and the settings on the unit itself. You'll feel cared for and confident knowing every detail has been fine-tuned just for you.

Finally, we'll explain how the table will move and what you might feel during the session. The Triton uses controlled, gentle movements to create traction or targeted decompression, depending on your treatment plan. Some patients say it feels like a light stretching sensation, while others describe it as soothing pressure relief. If at any point you feel uncomfortable, just let us know—we can adjust the settings or stop the process immediately.

The entire placement process is designed to make you feel safe, supported, and at ease. By the time your session starts, you'll be perfectly positioned to reap the benefits of this innovative treatment. Relax, take a deep breath, and look forward to feeling better!

The Triton is all about putting patient comfort first. Its ergonomic design keeps patients feeling supported and relaxed during therapy, while the smooth, gentle operation avoids the discomfort that often comes with traditional decompression methods. The easy-to-use interface makes quick adjustments simple, creating a seamless experience for both patients and practitioners. Every detail of the Triton has been carefully designed with patients in mind. From adaptable traction settings to its quiet, calming operation, the Triton helps create a soothing environment that builds trust and encourages relaxation. This focus on comfort not only keeps patients happy but also helps them stick to their treatment plans—key for getting real, long-term results. By making the whole process more positive and less intimidating, the Triton helps patients fully embrace their recovery journey.

The Triton goes beyond just basic functionality, addressing the bigger picture for both healthcare providers and patients. Its advanced technology is backed by solid scientific validation, ensuring every feature delivers real, measurable results. The device integrates effortlessly into existing clinical workflows, making it easy for practitioners to get started and focus on what really matters—providing great care. It also supports data tracking and reporting, letting providers monitor patient progress over time and adjust treatment plans as needed. This data-driven approach helps build stronger provider-patient relationships, giving patients clear proof of their progress and boosting trust in the treatment process. For clinics, the Triton isn't just new equipment—it's an investment in the future of patient-centered care.

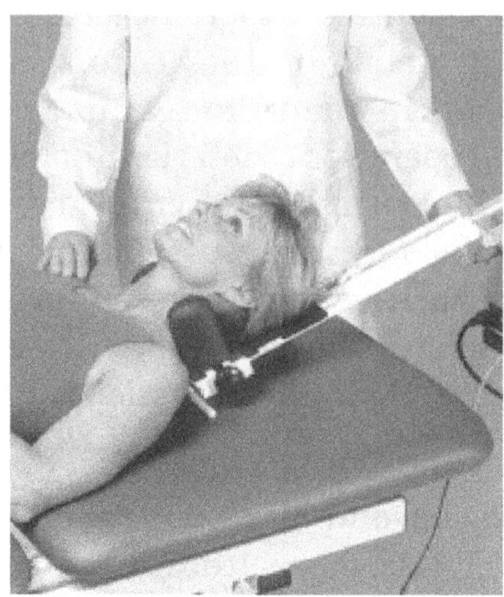

The Chattanooga Triton Decompression Unit is changing the game for non-surgical spinal care. This isn't just another device—it's a cutting-edge solution that's all about putting patients first. With its advanced technology and focus on comfort, the Triton sets a new standard for spinal decompression therapy. Each treatment is fully customized to meet the unique needs of every patient, ensuring the best possible results.

What really makes the Triton special is how it benefits both patients and practitioners. For patients, it offers real relief from chronic back pain and spinal issues that might have felt impossible to overcome. It helps people get back to their daily lives with less pain and more confidence. For practitioners, it's a reliable, easy-to-use tool that streamlines treatments, saves time, and delivers amazing results. It's a win-win that builds trust and improves the overall care experience.

The Triton isn't just about treating pain—it's about transforming lives. Patients can look forward to living more active, fulfilling lives without being held back by spinal discomfort. In a world where medical technology keeps evolving, the Triton stands out as a leader—smart, effective, and truly patient-focused. For any practitioner wanting to deliver innovative and efficient care, the Triton isn't just a tool—it's a total game-changer. With the Triton, relief is more than possible—it's life-changing.

Chapter 6
Glucosamine Sulfate, Glycosaminoglycans, and Their Role in Disc Health and Joint Healing

The human body's ability to heal and regenerate is truly amazing. One of the most important processes is the repair and maintenance of cartilage and connective tissues, which are essential for keeping us mobile and reducing pain, especially in the spine and major joints. At the heart of this process are glucosamine sulfate and glycosaminoglycans (GAGs)—two key players that help keep cartilage and intervertebral discs healthy, hydrated, and able to handle stress. By supporting cartilage repair and improving hydration, these compounds can make a big difference in managing arthritis, injuries, and spinal health issues. When paired with traction therapy—a technique that uses negative pressure to draw nutrients into the discs—their benefits can become even more effective.

This chapter dives into how glucosamine sulfate and glycosaminoglycans repair connective tissues and how traction therapy helps distribute these compounds. By exploring their mechanisms, uses, and benefits, this approach gives hope to those looking for non-invasive ways to improve joint and spinal health.

Glucosamine Sulfate's Essential Role in Cartilage Health

Glucosamine sulfate is a naturally occurring compound found in the body, primarily within cartilage. It serves as a precursor to glycosaminoglycans, the molecules responsible for forming the structural framework of cartilage, ligaments, and intervertebral discs. Think of glucosamine sulfate as the raw material necessary for producing GAGs. Without it, the body struggles to maintain the health and elasticity of cartilage and connective tissues.

Cartilage is crucial for its shock-absorbing and lubricating properties, particularly in weight-bearing joints like the knees and hips, as well as in the intervertebral discs of the spine, which cushion vertebrae against the forces of daily movement. Over time, however, wear and tear, injuries, or degenerative conditions such as arthritis or disc disease can deplete the body's natural supply of glucosamine sulfate. This leads to reduced glycosaminoglycan production, causing cartilage to thin and lose its ability to retain water. The outcome? Pain, inflammation, and diminished mobility.

Glucosamine supplementation aims to replenish this supply, kick-starting the regeneration of GAGs. Clinical research shows that glucosamine sulfate may help reduce symptoms of osteoarthritis, particularly in the knees, by slowing cartilage degradation and supporting repair. Although its effects may take several weeks to manifest, many patients report lasting relief and improved joint function when it is used consistently.

Understanding Glycosaminoglycans (GAGs) and Their Impact

Glycosaminoglycans, often referred to as the foundational molecules of joint and disc health, are long chains of sugar molecules that provide critical structural and functional support to connective tissues. There are several types of GAGs, including:

- **Glucosamine sulfate** – Most abundant and plays a pivotal role in the body's ability to synthesize glycosaminoglycans.
- **Chondroitin sulfate** – Known for its ability to

> resist compression, chondroitin sulfate is integral to cartilage resilience.
> - **Hyaluronic acid** – Plays a vital role in tissue hydration and lubrication, particularly within synovial fluid in joints.
> - **Keratan sulfate** – Found in cartilage and spinal discs, contributing to mechanical strength and integrity.

The primary role of GAGs is to attract and retain water in the cartilage and intervertebral discs. This hydration is essential because it gives these tissues their unique elasticity and ability to endure physical stress. Under healthy conditions, GAGs enable cartilage and discs to act like sponges, compressing and decompressing in response to movement while maintaining structural integrity. However, when GAG levels decline, tissues become brittle, and cracks appear, setting the stage for chronic pain and dysfunction.

One of the most significant impacts of GAGs is their ability to support the nucleus pulposus—the gel-like core of intervertebral discs. The nucleus relies on water retention for its shock-absorbing abilities, and GAGs play a vital role in sustaining this hydration. Ensuring a steady supply of GAGs through supplementation with glucosamine sulfate becomes even more critical when the natural aging process or injury compromises disc health.

Glucosamine Sulfate: The Essential Building Block

Glucosamine sulfate plays a pivotal role in the body's ability to synthesize glycosaminoglycans (GAGs), which are essential macromolecules found in the extracellular matrix of connective tissues. As the rate-limiting substrate, if there is enough glucosamine sulfate in the body, it can produce all other GAGs. These GAGs, such as chondroitin sulfate, keratan sulfate, and heparan sulfate, are crucial for maintaining the structural integrity and function of cartilage, ligaments, and tendons. The availability of glucosamine sulfate ensures that the body has the necessary building blocks to maintain healthy joint function and repair damaged tissues.

Despite the body's capacity to produce some glucosamine naturally, its synthesis can be insufficient, particularly as individuals age or experience increased joint stress. Supplementing with glucosamine sulfate can support the body's ability to maintain adequate GAG levels, thereby promoting better joint health and mobility. Unlike other GAGs, which require glucosamine for their production, glucosamine sulfate acts as a precursor that enables the synthesis of other essential GAGs. This pathway emphasizes the importance of glucosamine sulfate in joint health, as it is directly tied to the biosynthesis of the compounds that provide cartilage with its shock-absorbing and lubricating properties.

The unique role of glucosamine sulfate as a rate-limiting GAG highlights its critical contribution to overall musculoskeletal health. By modulating the production of other GAGs, glucosamine sulfate ensures that connective tissues remain resilient and capable of withstanding daily wear and tear. For individuals looking to support their joint health, understanding this process underscores the potential benefits of incorporating glucosamine sulfate into their supplement regimen. This understanding encourages a proactive approach to maintaining joint vitality and function, allowing people to lead active and pain-free lives.

Arthritis and Acute Injuries: Repairing Damage with GAGs

Arthritis, particularly osteoarthritis, often involves the gradual breakdown of cartilage within joints. This erosion leads to bones rubbing against each other, causing pain, inflammation, and stiffness. Similarly, acute injuries—such as ligament tears or joint trauma—can disrupt the integrity of connective tissues, slowing recovery. Chronic conditions and acute damage share a common feature—the need for glycosaminoglycans to facilitate repair.

Studies have demonstrated that glucosamine sulfate supplementation can stimulate glycosaminoglycan production, promoting cartilage repair. It helps chondrocytes, the cells responsible for cartilage maintenance, increase their output of chondroitin sulfate and other GAGs. Over time, this not only alleviates the symptoms of arthritis but also enhances the healing process in injured joints by reducing inflammation and improving hydration in damaged tissues.

The Science Behind Traction Therapy and Nutrient Delivery

While glucosamine sulfate aids in glycosaminoglycan production, ensuring these crucial molecules reach the discs and cartilage is another challenge altogether. Intervertebral discs, for instance, are avascular structures, meaning they lack direct blood vessels for nutrient delivery. They rely on a process called diffusion, where nutrients from nearby blood vessels and endplates travel into the disc gradually. This process is often insufficient when the discs are dehydrated, degenerating, or under constant compression.

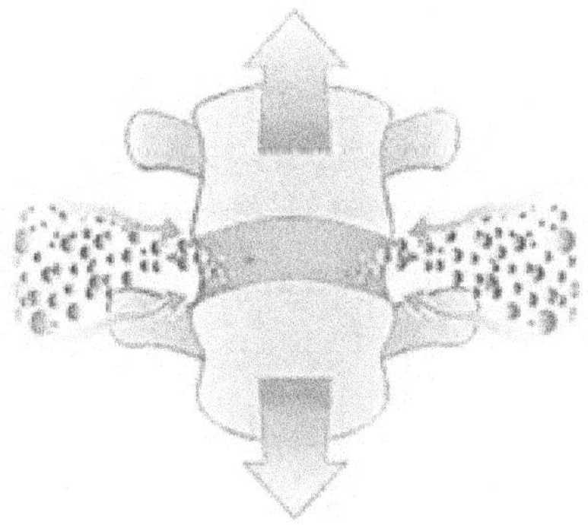

Traction therapy addresses this limitation by creating negative pressure within the intervertebral discs. This vacuum-like effect is achieved by gently stretching the spine using specialized traction tables or decompression devices. Negative pressure has two primary benefits:

1. **Rehydrating the Discs**: By reducing intradiscal pressure, traction therapy allows fluids, nutrients, and oxygen to move more efficiently into the disc's nucleus pulposus. This includes glycosaminoglycans, which are essential for reversing dehydration and restoring the disc's ability to absorb shocks.

2. **Relieving Pressure on Nerves**: When discs become herniated or bulge, they press against spinal nerves, resulting in pain, tingling, or numbness. Traction helps retract the disc material into its proper position, alleviating this nerve compression.

Patients undergoing traction therapy often report significant pain relief after several sessions, particularly when combined with interventions like glucosamine supplementation. Over time, the combined efforts of traction and glycosaminoglycans repair the biomechanical and metabolic deficits that contribute to disc deterioration.

Combining Treatments for

Maximum Benefit

The combination of glucosamine sulfate, glycosaminoglycans, and traction therapy exemplifies a holistic approach to healing that prioritizes natural restoration over invasive interventions. One case study illustrates this synergy:

Case Study

A 52-year-old patient with early-stage degenerative disc disease and knee osteoarthritis experienced chronic pain and limited mobility. A treatment plan combining daily glucosamine sulfate supplementation with biweekly spinal traction sessions was implemented over 12 weeks. By the end of the program, the patient reported increased spinal flexibility, reduced knee stiffness, and measurable improvements in disc hydration on imaging studies.

This success underscores the potential of integrative therapies to support long-term healing without the risks associated with surgery or prolonged use of painkillers.

Challenges and Considerations

While the benefits of glucosamine sulfate and traction therapy are clear, there are some challenges to consider:

- **Patience and Consistency**: Both treatments require time to produce noticeable effects. Patients should be counseled on setting realistic expectations and adhering to their regimen.
- **Variability in Response**: Not everyone responds equally to glucosamine supplementation or traction therapy. Factors such as age, severity of degeneration, and overall health can influence outcomes.
- **Supplement Quality**: The effectiveness of glucosamine sulfate depends on the purity and dosage of the

supplement. Patients should choose clinically tested products from reputable manufacturers.

Despite these challenges, the combination of glucosamine sulfate and traction therapy holds immense promise for addressing spine and joint health.

A Path Toward True Healing

Glucosamine sulfate and glycosaminoglycans are more than just molecules; they represent the body's natural tools for repair and resilience. Combined with modern traction therapy, they offer a safe, effective, and evidence-based approach to tackling arthritis, acute injuries, and disc issues at their root causes. By focusing on rehydrating tissues, reducing inflammation, and encouraging regeneration, these treatments provide hope to those seeking alternatives to surgery and medications.

The road to lasting recovery requires persistence, but the rewards—restored mobility, reduced pain, and a higher quality of life—are well worth the effort. With a deeper understanding of the science behind these natural and mechanical interventions, patients can step confidently into a future of better health.

Chapter 7
More Than Just Pain: Understanding the Mental and Emotional Impact of Chronic Pain

Living with chronic pain isn't just about physical discomfort. It changes how you experience life—how you move, how you sleep, how you interact with others, and even how you see yourself. When pain becomes a daily reality, especially from conditions like disc injuries or nerve compression, it's not just your body that suffers. The emotional and mental toll is just as real, and often, it's the part that goes unnoticed.

You start to feel disconnected from the things that once brought you joy—maybe it's an active lifestyle, playing with your kids, or even just sitting through a movie without shifting in discomfort every five minutes. The frustration builds. You're tired of explaining your pain to people who don't get it. You push through, but deep down, you wonder if this is just how life is going to be from now on. That kind of weight, carried over weeks, months, or even years, takes a toll far beyond the physical.

The Mind-Body Connection in Chronic Pain

Pain isn't just something you feel—it's something your brain processes. That means your emotional state, your stress levels, and your overall mental health all play a role in how intense your pain feels. If you've ever noticed that stress makes your pain worse, or that a good day with friends makes you feel a little lighter, that's the mind-body connection at work.

The tricky part is that chronic pain and emotional distress

feed off each other. Pain causes stress, stress makes pain feel worse, and before you know it, you're stuck in a cycle where both your physical and emotional well-being are suffering. Anxiety and depression often creep in—sometimes so subtly that you don't even realize it's happening. You start avoiding social plans, fearing that pain will get in the way. You feel like a burden. Over time, that isolation makes everything worse.

But here's the thing: pain is complex, and that means treatment needs to be just as comprehensive. Addressing the physical aspect alone isn't always enough—you need a full-body, full-mind approach.

The Role of Counseling in Pain Management

That's where counseling comes in. Seeking mental health support doesn't mean your pain isn't real or that it's "all in your head." It means you recognize that chronic pain affects every part of you, and you deserve care that reflects that reality.

At Curis Functional Health, we incorporate mental health support alongside chiropractic care, non-surgical spinal decompression, and functional medicine. Why? Because addressing pain means treating you as a whole person—not just focusing on the physical symptoms.

Counseling helps break the cycle of pain and emotional distress. Techniques like Cognitive Behavioral Therapy (CBT) can rewire negative thought patterns that make pain feel even worse. Mindfulness-Based Stress Reduction (MBSR) teaches you how to be present with your body without spiraling into fear about pain. Acceptance and Commitment Therapy (ACT) helps shift your focus from pain avoidance to living a fulfilling life, even when discomfort is part of the equation.

When you combine these approaches with treatments like non-surgical spinal decompression and chiropractic care, you're not just managing pain—you're changing how your body and mind respond to it.

Finding a Path Forward

If you've been living with chronic pain, I want you to hear this: you're not alone, and there are real solutions that don't just mask the symptoms. Pain doesn't have to define your life, and seeking support for your mental health is one of the most powerful steps you can take.

At Curis Functional Health Chicago Lakeview, we believe in treating the whole person—not just the symptoms. We blend cutting-edge physical treatments with functional wellness strategies and counseling, ensuring that patients don't just feel better temporarily, but actually get their lives back.

You deserve to move freely. You deserve to wake up without dread. You deserve relief. And we're here to help you find it.

Chapter 8
Caring for Your Spine Through Exercise

Taking care of your spine is one of the best things you can do for yourself, especially if you're dealing with disc degeneration or recovering from an injury. Movement is like medicine for your body. It helps reduce pain, strengthens the muscles that support your spine, and promotes healing. Even simple exercises can work wonders if you do them regularly and with care. The exercises we'll cover here are beginner-friendly, safe, and aimed at improving your spinal health. One method we'll talk more about is the McKenzie exercises, which have been specially designed for disc issues. But first, let's understand why these movements are so beneficial.

Exercise keeps your spine mobile and the surrounding muscles strong. This takes stress off damaged discs, helping to reduce pain and support recovery. It also improves circulation, which can help deliver much-needed nutrients to the injury site. Plus, the right exercises can improve your posture, which might help relieve pressure on problem areas. The key is to listen to your body—if something feels painful, stop and adjust. And before starting, always consult with your healthcare provider if you're unsure about what's safe for you.

Gentle Warm-Up

Now, before jumping into exercises, it's important to loosen up with a gentle warm-up. You don't need anything fancy here; even a quick walk or a few light stretches will do. Try rolling your shoulders or easing tension with some neck rolls. This prepares your body for movement, making the exercises feel smoother and more effective. Always start with a simple warm-up to give your muscles and joints a chance to wake up.

Once you feel warm and ready, you can move on to the following exercises:

Basic Exercises for Disc Health

Simple Movements for Spine Health

One of the best places to start is with basic exercises that ease tension and strengthen your core. Take the Cat-Cow stretch, for example. It's a simple movement where you arch and round your back in a flowing motion while on your hands and knees. Besides warming up your spine, it helps improve flexibility and can ease stiffness. Another great option is the pelvic tilt. While lying on your back, you gently flatten your lower back into the floor by engaging your core—this targets your abdominal muscles and reduces stress on your spine. If you're looking for something to relax and stretch your lower back, Child's Pose is worth trying. Just kneel down, stretch your arms out forward, and rest your forehead on the floor. It's a calming movement that feels great after a long day.

Below are the detailed steps to executing these exercises. These are gentle movements meant to strengthen your core, improve your spinal alignment, and to help with disc degeneration or injury.

1. Cat-Cow Stretch

- **Purpose**: Improves spine mobility and reduces stiffness.
- **How to Do It**:
    1. Start on your hands and knees in a tabletop position. Keep your wrists under your shoulders and your knees under your hips.

2. Begin by inhaling as you arch your back, lifting your head and tailbone toward the ceiling (this is the "Cow" position).
3. Next, exhale as you round your back, tucking your chin to your chest and tailbone under (this is the "Cat" position).
4. Alternate between Cat and Cow for 5-10 repetitions, moving slowly and gently.

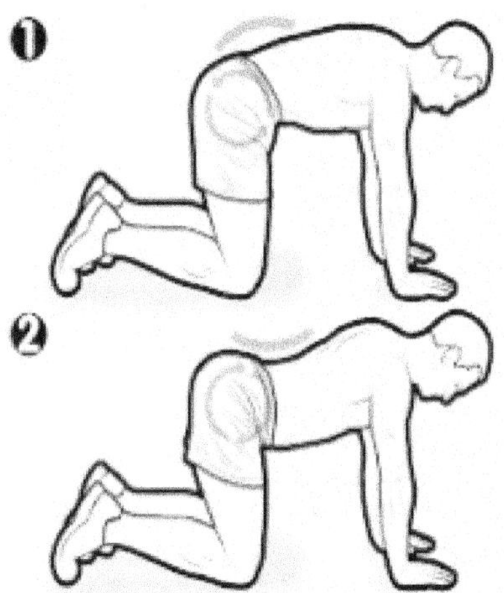

2. Pelvic Tilt

- **Purpose**: Strengthens the core and reduces lower back pressure.
- **How to Do It**:
  1. Lie on your back with your knees bent and your feet flat on the floor, about hip-width apart.
  2. Flatten your lower back onto the floor by tilting your pelvis upward (as if pulling your belly button toward your spine).
  3. Hold for 3-5 seconds, then release.
  4. Repeat for 10-12 repetitions.

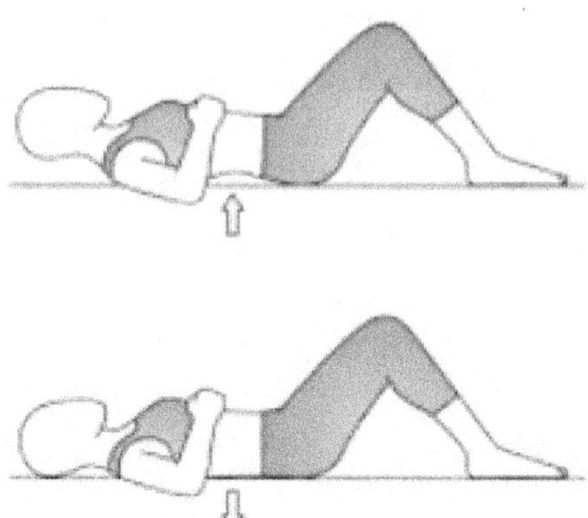

3. Child's Pose

- **Purpose**: Stretches the lower back and hips while promoting relaxation.
- **How to Do It**:
  1. Start by kneeling on the floor and sitting back on your heels.
  2. Slowly reach your arms forward, lowering your chest toward the ground.
  3. Rest your forehead on the mat and take deep breaths.
  4. Hold this position for 20-30 seconds, then release. Repeat 2-3 times.

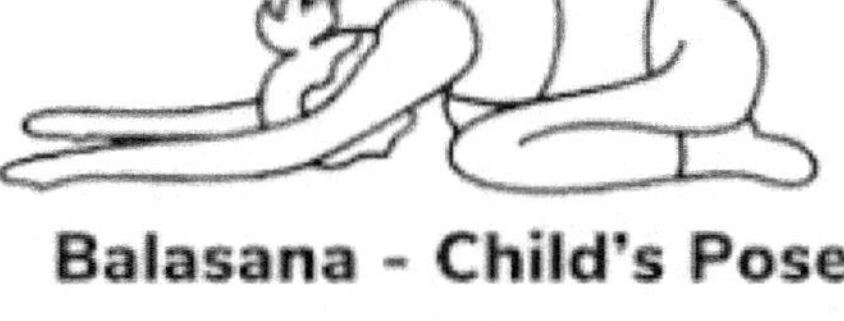

Understanding McKenzie Exercises and Their Benefits

McKenzie exercises, or the McKenzie Method of Mechanical Diagnosis and Therapy (MDT), are a series of targeted movements designed to improve spinal health, particularly for those dealing with disc issues like herniation, degeneration, or sciatica. This method was developed by physical therapist Robin McKenzie in the 1950s and has since become widely recognized for its effectiveness in managing back and neck pain. These exercises aim to reduce pressure on spinal discs, promote proper alignment, and alleviate nerve compression through simple, controlled movements.

The key principle behind McKenzie Exercises is that certain repeated movements and sustained positions can help centralize pain. This means that instead of radiating down the legs or into the arms, as is often the case with disc injuries, the pain moves closer to the spine and becomes more localized. This shift is considered a positive response, as it usually signals improvement and a reduction in nerve irritation.

The Benefits of McKenzie Exercises

The McKenzie Method is valued for its simplicity and adaptability. The exercises can be tailored to each individual's condition and are designed to empower patients to manage their symptoms independently. Here are some of the key benefits of McKenzie Exercises:

1. Reduced Disc Pressure

By encouraging proper spinal extension and alignment, McKenzie exercises help relieve pressure on bulging or herniated discs. This not only alleviates pain but can also prevent further damage over time.

2. Improved Mobility and Flexibility

These exercises restore the spine's natural range of motion by gently stretching and moving it in specific directions. This can help reduce stiffness and make everyday movements easier.

3. Pain Relief

Many McKenzie movements provide immediate relief by decompressing nerves and reducing inflammation around problem areas. Over time, consistent practice can lead to sustained symptom reduction.

What Research Says

The McKenzie Method has been the subject of various scientific studies, and its effectiveness is well-documented in the realm of conservative treatment for back pain, lumbar disc herniation or sciatica.

For instance, a review of clinical studies has shown that McKenzie Exercises effectively reduce lower back pain intensity and improve overall function compared to other standard treatments. One study even found that patients practicing the McKenzie Method experienced faster symptom relief than those following general physical therapy routines.

Research has also highlighted the McKenzie Method's ability

to centralize pain, which is associated with better recovery outcomes. Healthcare professionals frequently recommend these exercises because they are non-invasive, require no equipment, and pose minimal risk when performed correctly.

Why Healthcare Professionals Endorse McKenzie

The McKenzie Method aligns with best practices in spinal health care because it prioritizes patient empowerment and self-care. Doctors, physical therapists, and chiropractors appreciate how the exercises encourage patients to actively participate in their recovery process. This active approach reduces reliance on medications or invasive treatments like surgery in many cases.

If you've been advised to try McKenzie exercises, it's a sign that your provider sees value in a strategy built around improving spinal mechanics naturally. Always work with a professional to ensure you're performing the exercises correctly, especially when starting out. With consistent practice, McKenzie movements can be an incredibly effective tool for managing spinal pain and improving your overall quality of life.

The Power of McKenzie Exercises

For anyone dealing with more serious disc issues, the McKenzie exercises can be a game-changer. They're designed to help with bulging or herniated discs by encouraging proper spinal alignment, and many people find they also relieve sciatica or similar pain. We'll start with the simplest one, called Prone Lying. You just lie on your stomach, letting your lower back relax for a minute or two. That's it. Even this simple step can gently ease pressure in your back.

Building on that is Prone Props, where you begin lying on your stomach and then prop yourself up onto your elbows, keeping your hips on the ground. This is excellent for re-aligning the spine and relieving nerve compression. Stay in this position for ten seconds at first, gradually working your way up to longer holds as you feel more comfortable. Finally, there's the Standing Extension. This one's great for quick relief, especially if you've been sitting for too long. All you do is stand with your hands on your lower back for support and gently arch backward. It's quick, easy, and often effective for releasing pressure.

When doing McKenzie exercises, the key is consistency. These movements should be painless, so be mindful of your limits and go slow, especially at first. Regular practice can make a significant difference in reducing pain and improving your mobility over time.

1. Prone Lying

- **Purpose**: Begins the process of easing pressure in the lower back.

- **How to Do It**:

    1. Lie face down on a flat surface, like the floor. Place a pillow under your chest if this feels more comfortable.

    2. Rest your arms at your sides and keep your neck in a neutral position.

    3. Stay in this position for 1-2 minutes, breathing deeply and allowing your lower back to relax.

2. Prone Props (Extension in Lying)

- **Purpose**: Helps to reverse disc bulging and reduce nerve compression.

- **How to Do It**:

    1. Start lying face down as in the prone lying

position.

2. Slowly prop yourself up onto your elbows, keeping your hips pressed to the ground.

3. Hold this position for 10-15 seconds, then lower back down.

4. Repeat 6-8 times, gradually increasing the time you stay propped up as it becomes more comfortable.

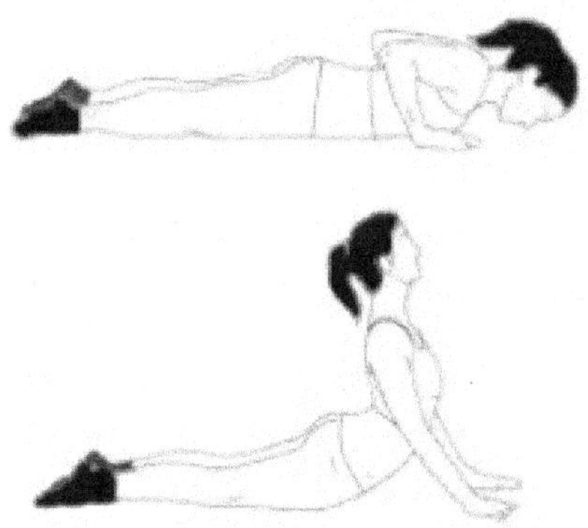

3. Standing Extension

- **Purpose**: Provides quick relief for low back pain, especially after sitting for long periods.

- **How to Do It**:

    1. Stand with your feet about hip-width apart and place your hands on your lower back for support.

    2. Gently lean slightly backward, extending your spine.

3. Hold for 2-3 seconds, then return to neutral.

4. Repeat up to 10 times.

Embrace Your Journey to Spinal Health

Taking care of your spine can feel like a big challenge, especially when you're dealing with disc degeneration or an injury. But here's the good news: gentle, consistent exercises can make a real difference in easing your pain and helping you move more freely. The moves we've gone over, especially the McKenzie Exercises, aren't complicated, but they're powerful tools to help strengthen your spine and support healing.

The key is to focus on progress, not perfection. Start slow, pay attention to what feels right for your body, and celebrate every bit of improvement, no matter how small it seems. Consistency is everything, so try to make these exercises part of your daily routine—it's an investment in your long-term health.

Remember, you don't have to do this alone. Check in with your healthcare provider before kicking off a new routine to make sure it's a good fit for you. They can provide guidance and adjustments to ensure you're on the right track. Now, set aside a few minutes each day to show your spine some love—you've got this!

Chapter 9
Success Stories: Inspiring Case Studies of Disc Recovery and Healing

Sarah's Journey to Recovery from Severe Sciatica

Pain was a constant companion for Sarah. At just 39 years old, her life as a passionate teacher had taken a dramatic turn. The searing ache in her lower back radiates down her right leg, making every step feel like an exercise in endurance. Tasks as simple as bending to tie her shoes or demonstrating a lesson for her students became excruciating. For Sarah, the words "lumbar disc herniation at L5-S1" felt both daunting and mysterious. Added to this was a compressed nerve triggering the dreaded symptoms of sciatica. Her medical doctors presented surgery as a likely solution, listing out the risks and recovery timelines. But Sarah wasn't ready to surrender to the operating table. What she sought instead was relief—without sacrificing her long-term health.

Sarah's first chiropractic visit was filled with a mix of hope and apprehension. I reviewed her imaging, explaining how the integrative approach she would adopt could work. "We'll begin by addressing your pelvis," I described. "A subtle tilt there is throwing off the alignment of your lumbar spine, which is likely adding stress to the affected area." Over the weeks, gentle yet precise adjustments began correcting that imbalance. During her second phase of care, Sarah undertook non-surgical spinal decompression therapy. Lying on a specialized table, she experienced a controlled stretch to her spine, which alleviated some of the pressure almost immediately. The negative pressure generated by this traction encouraged hydration, reduced inflammation, and worked to "vacuum" the bulging herniated material back into place.

The third component of Sarah's treatment plan was glucosamine sulfate. I thoroughly explained its role. "Think of this as nourishment for your damaged disc," I shared. "It helps your body produce glycosaminoglycans, which attract water and give discs their shock-absorbing qualities."

Over the next weeks, Sarah remained committed to the program. There were ups and downs; some days felt like setbacks when long hours of sitting robbed her of relief. She decided the final step in her healing was to add counseling sessions to help her emotionally as well. With talk therapy as well as guided meditations, she slowly improved and her persistence paid off.

By the end of three months, Sarah's pain levels had decreased dramatically. A follow-up imaging confirmed what her body already told her—the herniation had shrunk significantly. Once again, teaching became a joy rather than an obstacle. For Sarah, the most empowering realization was not just the absence of pain, but the knowledge that her body—when given the right care—was fully capable of healing.

Fighting Degeneration: Michael's Regaining of Motion in His Golden Years

Michael shuffled into the clinic, shoulders slumped and expression resigned. At 62, he had lived with degenerative disc disease for nearly a decade. Within the past year, however, his condition had worsened, bringing chronic aching pain and stiffness in his lower back. Morning walks he used to cherish dwindled as bending or sitting down for longer than a minute became unbearable. X-ray imaging showed thinning, dehydrated discs particularly at L3-L4 and L4-L5, robbing them of their cushioning qualities. Traditional treatments had brought temporary relief, but Michael didn't want to rely on medications or pursue surgery. Instead, he sought something more restorative.

Michael presented to my office and after a thorough and detailed exam and consultation, he was set up on a concise treatment plan, targeting his stiff lumbar spine through adjustments that gently improved mobility. Though subtle, these changes removed vertebral restrictions that were aggravating the pain. Chiropractic care was paired with spinal decompression treatments. Using a decompression table, Michael's lumbar spine underwent carefully controlled stretching, creating the negative pressure needed to relieve irritated discs. Over time, this encouraged nutrients and fluids back into the discs, increasing their volume and pliability. At the same time, Michael began taking a daily glucosamine sulfate supplement. I explained how this compound supported his body's ability to make glycosaminoglycans—the essential building blocks of hydrated, healthy discs.

At first, progress was slow, which made Michael skeptical. But around his second month of care, he began noticing changes. Stiff mornings became manageable, his posture improved, and he was able to join his wife on short evening walks. By the three-month mark, Michael's pain had reduced by over 80%, and spine imaging revealed modest but meaningful improvements in his disc hydration and spacing. His newfound mobility lifted both his spirits and his confidence in aging actively. He could not believe how the chronic pain had put a damper on his happiness and sense of peace.

Michael ultimately credited his recovery to not only the physical healing but the emotional reassurance he gained. "For once, I felt like the people treating me were working with my body, not against it," he said, reflecting the optimism he now carried on his daily strolls.

Finding Relief After Years of Desk Work:

Lisa's Battle with a Cervical Bulge

For Lisa, the pain started in her neck—a dull ache that quietly crept in after long hours working at her desk. At 47, she barely noticed the signs at first. A faint stiffness would linger after meetings until one day it burst into sharp pain, accompanied by a numbing sensation running down her left arm. When the symptoms became too disruptive to ignore, she sought out a medical doctor and received her diagnosis. Lisa had a disc bulge at the C5-C6 level, causing compression on her nerves. Her medical doctor suggested surgery as a possible future course, but Lisa hesitated to take such a serious step. Feeling desperate, she researched alternative solutions, eventually stumbling upon the combined approach of chiropractic care and spinal decompression.

Lisa's treatment aimed to tackle the problem from every angle. Chiropractic manipulations targeted her cervical vertebrae and upper back, slowly restoring better alignment to her spine and shoulders. The decompression therapy utilized a specialized cervical traction device that gently stretched and opened her compressed area, relieving nerve impingement responsible for her arm numbness. Each session started to carry a sense of relief, and for the first time in months, Lisa looked forward to movement. Her at-home care included daily glucosamine sulfate and omega-3 fatty acid intake to decrease inflammation and boost disc repair.

One thing Lisa had overlooked in the past is her tendency to be a "workaholic." She decided to address this with some one on one counseling. Looking and working on her long-standing patterns of people pleasing helped her finally put herself and her healing first, while learning to trust that the job is still getting done.

Over weeks, the pain and tingling improved. Lisa recalled one particular morning when she woke up—and for the first time in months—she turned her head without grimacing or feeling constrained. By the end of her treatment plan, her numbness had disappeared completely, and she resumed her desk work with ergonomic changes in place. In the future, with proper care, she had not only healed physically but redefined her approach to self-care after years of overworking herself.

James' Athletic Comeback

James was no stranger to sports injuries. Soccer defined his life, first as a player and later as a coach. By 30, however, recurring lower back pain began interfering with him both on and off the field. His MRI showed a repeated herniation at L4-L5, which explained the frequent muscle spasms and shooting pains he experienced after routine scrimmages. Physical therapy helped strengthen his core muscles but didn't solve the root cause. That's when James decided to try an integrative plan at Curis Functional Health.

The chiropractic sessions focused on restoring proper alignment to his pelvis and lower back. Since James played and coached actively, correcting the subtle imbalances in his gait was essential. He underwent spinal decompression therapy, lying motionless on the table as the machine gently pulled and relaxed his lower back. This negative pressure encouraged his disc material to retract and allowed fluid and nutrients to penetrate his damaged disc. Alongside this, he began taking high-dose glucosamine supplements paired with collagen protein to strengthen connective tissues weakened by his athletic lifestyle.

Three months later, the results were undeniable. His herniated disc showed real signs of recovery on imaging, and his movements on the field became agile again. James didn't just regain his ability to coach; he found himself playing alongside his team with confidence and the power he thought he'd lost. Emotionally he never has felt more fulfilled. His recovery emphasized to him the importance of maintenance, regular body alignment, and long-term nutritional strategies.

Mary's Multi-Level Healing

For Mary, her career as a nurse demanded large physical and mental reserves. Decades of long shifts, heavy lifting, and minimal rest had taken a toll on her body, leaving her with bulging discs in both her cervical and lumbar spine. She experienced stiffness in her lower back, while shooting neck pain made day-to-day tasks unbearable. At 55, her body felt worn out beyond her years.

Mary began her care with consistent chiropractic adjustments targeting both problem areas of her spine. Alternating between cervical and lumbar decompression therapy, her sessions relieved the crushing pressure on her discs. At home, glucosamine sulfate paired with vitamin C helped supply her with the building blocks for healing—and after several weeks, her pain lessened noticeably.

Twelve weeks into her personalized treatment plan, Mary could turn her neck freely for the first time in years. Her back stiffness also eased, allowing her to finish shifts without collapsing in pain afterward. For Mary, the outcome wasn't just a physical transformation but one full of gratitude. She regained her mobility, her career energy, and an optimism she hadn't felt in over a decade.

A Shared Path to Healing

Each patient's story carried unique struggles and triumphs. Yet, the consistent thread among them was the integrative approach that prioritized healing both structurally and nutritionally. Chiropractic adjustments restored alignment, decompression reversed damage, some help to improve emotionally and glucosamine sulfate nourished recovery from within. These tools turned pain into empowerment, showing that with the right resources, support, and a focus on personal growth, people can tackle even the toughest challenges. This journey proves just how powerful resilience can be and how much healing is possible when folks have the tools they need to thrive.

Chapter 10
Hidden Dangers of Spinal Surgery, Failed Back Syndrome, and Opiates —and How Spinal Decompression Offers a Safer Solution

Dealing with the pain from disc injuries or degeneration can be overwhelming, affecting everything from your work to your daily activities and even your sleep. It often feels like the only options are risky surgeries or relying on painkillers like opiates. While these treatments might offer quick relief, they come with serious risks, including dependency, side effects, and long-term health consequences that can add to the burden. The good news? There's a safer, non-invasive option that targets the root cause of the pain without those major downsides. Spinal decompression therapy is a gentle, innovative treatment designed to relieve pressure on your spinal discs, promoting natural healing and reducing pain over time. It offers a path to recovery that lets you get back to living your life—free from harsh side effects, invasive procedures, or compromises.

The Risks of Spinal Surgery

Spinal surgery is often presented as a last resort for persistent cases of disc herniation, spinal stenosis, or degenerative disc disease. The goal of these procedures—such as a discectomy, laminectomy, or spinal fusion—is to correct spinal abnormalities, stabilize the spine, or relieve pressure on nerves. However, surgery comes with significant risks that are often underestimated.

Post-operative complications can include infections, blood clots, excessive bleeding, or nerve damage, which can lead to numbness or even paralysis. The process of recovering from spinal surgery is often long and grueling, requiring careful rehabilitation to regain mobility—if it is regained at all.

Among the most concerning outcomes is Failed Back Syndrome (FBS), a condition defined by persistent or worsening pain following spinal surgery. FBS occurs for a variety of reasons, including surgical complications, nerve damage, scar tissue buildup, or an improper diagnosis of the original issue. Imagine undergoing a complex surgical procedure, enduring weeks or months of recovery, only to find yourself trapped in a cycle of unrelenting pain.

Spinal fusion, one of the most common surgeries for degenerative disc disease, carries unique risks. While it may stabilize the spine by fusing two vertebrae together, this process shifts additional stress onto adjacent vertebrae, leading to a condition known as adjacent segment degeneration. Over time, this added strain increases the likelihood of further disc issues, often necessitating additional surgeries. Each subsequent operation amplifies the risks, creating a downward spiral of medical interventions that leave patients both physically and emotionally drained.

The Danger of Opiates and Painkillers

Many individuals experiencing spinal pain turn to opiates and painkillers for immediate relief. While medications like oxycodone and hydrocodone can temporarily mask pain, their long-term use is fraught with risks that extend beyond physical health.

Opiates are profoundly addictive, altering brain chemistry and causing dependency with sustained use. This tolerance forces individuals to escalate their dosage to achieve the same level of relief. The result? A devastating cycle of addiction that exacerbates the original problem without addressing its cause.

According to public health data, thousands of people every year find themselves battling opioid addiction indirectly caused by pain management practices.

Beyond addiction, prolonged use of opiates can suppress natural pain response mechanisms, impair cognitive function, and create severe gastrointestinal issues, including chronic constipation. Meanwhile, their effectiveness diminishes over time, and their role as a mere "band-aid" for deeper structural problems becomes apparent.

Non-opiates like NSAIDs (non-steroidal anti-inflammatory drugs), too, are not without their risks. Medications such as ibuprofen and naproxen can irritate the stomach lining, leading to ulcers and, in severe cases, significant gastrointestinal bleeding. Regular use of NSAIDs has also been associated with kidney damage and an increased risk of cardiovascular issues.

The Promise of Spinal Decompression Therapy

Given the pitfalls of surgery and medications, spinal decompression therapy stands out as a safer, non-invasive alternative that directly addresses the root causes of disc injury and degeneration. Unlike temporary fixes or drastic surgical measures, decompression therapy aims to restore balance and health to the spine, alleviating pain at its source.

Spinal decompression therapy gently stretches the spine using a specialized, motorized traction table. This process achieves two critical outcomes. First, it reduces pressure within the vertebral discs by creating a vacuum-like negative pressure. This action helps retract problematic disc material—such as herniations or bulging tissue—back into its proper position. Essentially, it's like reversing the process that initially caused the disc injury.

Second, the negative pressure encourages nutrient-rich fluids, oxygen, and healing substances to flow back into the discs. These intervertebral discs are largely avascular, meaning they lack a strong blood supply. This natural infusion of nutrients enhances the body's ability to repair and regenerate damaged tissue, reducing inflammation and restoring optimal disc function over time.

Why Decompression is a Safer Alternative

Spinal decompression therapy offers several advantages over traditional methods of addressing spinal issues. Most notably, it is **non-invasive**, eliminating the risks associated with surgery, such as infections or complications from anesthesia. Patients undergoing decompression therapy experience no incisions, no recovery downtime, and no need for potentially harmful medications.

Unlike painkillers, which only mask symptoms without addressing underlying structural problems, decompression therapy works to correct the root cause of disc-related issues. For example, in the case of a bulging or herniated disc, decompression effectively redistributes pressure in the spine, helping the disc material return to its proper configuration.

Preliminary studies and patient testimonials often describe an improvement in pain after only a handful of decompression sessions. For many, these results are long-lasting, providing relief that was previously thought unattainable without invasive surgery.

Real-Life Applications of Decompression

For someone suffering from chronic lower back pain due to degenerative disc disease, the burden often feels insurmountable. Surgery might seem inevitable, and painkillers—while tempting —can only offer fleeting relief. However, decompression therapy can dramatically reduce symptoms by enhancing the integrity of the spine's structural components.

A 48-year-old office worker, for example, who spends most of their day seated, might experience lumbar disk herniation from prolonged periods of poor posture. Instead of succumbing to surgery or struggling with the side effects of NSAIDs, regular decompression treatments can mitigate this pressure, restore proper alignment, and even prevent future disc deterioration.

Another common scenario involves athletes who endure repetitive spinal strain from high-impact sports. Here too, decompression therapy serves as both a treatment and preventive measure, offering relief while allowing the body to naturally repair itself.

A Proactive Approach to Spinal Health

Aside from decompression therapy, emphasizing spinal health through preventive measures is essential to maintaining long-term comfort and mobility. Maintaining a healthy weight, strengthening core muscles, and practicing good posture all contribute to reducing strain on the spine. Regular low-impact exercises such as yoga or swimming can further protect against degeneration and injury.

When combined with spinal decompression therapy, these lifestyle adjustments create a holistic program for spinal wellness. They not only mitigate existing pain but also prevent the recurrence of issues that often consign individuals to a cycle of surgeries and medications.

Reclaiming Life Through Natural Healing

Spinal decompression offers a path forward for those burdened by the perils of surgery and pharmaceutical dependency. By addressing the root causes of disc injuries and degeneration, decompression therapy empowers patients to reimagine their relationship with chronic pain.

Rather than resorting to invasive surgeries with uncertain outcomes or navigating the treacherous waters of opioid dependency, decompression provides a clear, non-invasive, and scientifically sound solution. It delivers not just relief, but also the opportunity to reclaim agency over one's health and well-being.

For anyone considering their options for spinal care, it's time to explore decompression therapy—not as a last-ditch effort, but as a first choice that offers safe, effective, and evidence-backed results. Through patience and consistency, many are finding it to be the key to leading pain-free, revitalized lives.

Chapter 11
A Detailed Review of Research on Chiropractic Care, Non-Surgical Spinal Decompression, Glycosaminoglycans, Emotional Impact and Alternative Solutions for Failed Back Surgery and Opiate Addiction

Chronic back injuries can lead to more than just physical pain—they often take a toll on emotional, social, and mental well-being, too. One particularly troubling issue linked to back pain is the increased risk of opioid abuse. Many people with unresolved back injuries are prescribed opioids to manage their pain, but what starts as a short-term fix can quickly turn into long-term dependency. This not only lowers quality of life but also creates new health problems.

This section explores the connection between back injuries and opioid abuse, highlighting research that reveals how pain management can sometimes lead to addiction. Through clinical studies, expert insights, and real-life cases, it's clear that finding alternative, non-invasive ways to manage pain is more important than ever.

The Escalation From Pain Management to Dependency

Opiate medications are frequently prescribed for patients experiencing severe and chronic back pain due to herniated discs, bulging discs, degenerative disc disease, or failed back surgery syndrome (FBSS). These medications, including hydrocodone, oxycodone, and morphine, provide a temporary reprieve from pain by binding to opioid receptors in the brain and spinal cord to block pain signals.

Studies Highlighting Opiate Usage in Back Pain:

1. **Journal of the American Medical Association (JAMA) Study**
   - **Title**: "Prescription Opioid Use in the Management of Chronic Non-Cancer Pain"
   - **Summary**: This longitudinal study reviewed 2,892 patients with chronic back pain prescribed opioids. Within 12 months, 21% of patients exhibited signs of dependency. The research emphasized the risk posed when addressing long-term pain with short-term medications.
   - **Published By**: *JAMA Internal Medicine*, 2015
2. **Pain Medicine Journal Meta-Analysis**
   - **Title**: "Chronic Pain Management and the Risk of Opioid Dependency in Spinal Disorders"
   - **Summary**: Analyzed 24 trials—including over 10,000 patients with back injuries treated with opioids. Findings showed a 68% increase in dependency rates versus patients using alternative therapies. This reinforces the risk opioids pose for patients with recurrent or unresolved pain conditions.
   - **Published By**: *Pain Medicine Journal*, 2018
3. **The Opioid Epidemic and Spinal Injuries**
   - A study conducted by the CDC revealed that individuals with chronic lower back pain are significantly more likely to receive opioid prescriptions, and 43% of these patients transitioned into misuse or addiction within two

years.
- **Source**: Centers for Disease Control and Prevention (CDC), 2019

The Biological and Psychological Mechanisms of Dependency

Physiologically, long-term use of opioids alters the brain's reward system, making it increasingly difficult for patients to manage pain without continued use of the medication. Simultaneously, psychological dependence arises as patients rely on opioids to function and mitigate their pain-induced anxiety. Research has also highlighted the heightened risk of tolerance, requiring escalating doses for the same level of relief, further increasing the risk of addiction.

Opioid Usage in Failed Back Surgery Syndrome (FBSS)

Failed Back Surgery Syndrome (FBSS) presents a unique challenge in managing chronic back pain. After unsuccessful surgical interventions, many patients still experience pain, leaving them vulnerable to opioid prescriptions as a last-resort option.

Supporting Evidence from Clinical Research:

1. **Journal of Neurosurgery Study on FBSS**
   - **Title**: "Assessing Opioid Dependency in Post-Surgical Spinal Patients"
   - **Summary**: This 2021 study followed FBSS patients prescribed opioids for ongoing pain management. Results showed that 63% of individuals developed dependency within three months, and only 14% reported satisfactory pain relief without

experiencing adverse effects.
- **Published By**: *Journal of Neurosurgery*, 2021
2. **Expert Analysis by Dr. Michael Freidman**
   - Dr. Friedman's comprehensive review described how FBSS patients turn to increasingly potent medications after spinal correction surgeries fail to yield results. He correlated opioid dependency with worsening physical mobility and psychological stress due to heightened pain sensitivity.
   - **Published By**: *Current Pain and Headache Reports*, 2020

The Limitations of Opioids in Managing Chronic Pain

Experts broadly agree that while opioids can temporarily alleviate severe pain, their long-term efficacy in chronic pain conditions is limited. The *Annals of Internal Medicine* (2019) published a landmark study showing no significant difference between opioid use and non-opioid alternatives (e.g., acetaminophen, NSAIDs) in terms of long-term back pain relief, but with significantly higher risks of adverse outcomes for opioid users.

Strategies for Non-Invasive Pain Management as Alternatives to Opioids

Given the risks highlighted, the integration of alternative, non-invasive therapies such as chiropractic care, non-surgical spinal decompression, and GAG supplementation is critical in breaking the cycle of opioid dependency.

1. **Chiropractic and Pain Relief**
   Research shows that patients who pursue chiropractic care report lower dependency on medications. A study in *Complementary Therapies in Medicine* revealed a 56%

reduction in painkiller use in chronic back pain patients over a six-month chiropractic treatment program.

2. **Spinal Decompression Therapy**

By targeting the source of the pain, such as herniated discs, decompression therapy provides long-term relief without pharmaceutical intervention. This was supported by a 2018 review from the *Journal of Pain Research*, which showed decompression therapy achieved sustained pain relief in 82% of patients previously reliant on opioids.

3. **Nutritional Support with GAGs**

Supplements like glucosamine and chondroitin actively support disc hydration and elasticity, reducing degeneration-related pain that often drives patients to seek opioids. Combined therapy using non-invasive solutions, as discussed throughout this book, proves more effective for long-term results than pharmacological pain management alone.

The Psychological Component in Recovery

Non-invasive treatments also address the psychological burden of chronic pain. Patients using therapies like chiropractic care or decompression frequently report improved quality of life and emotional well-being, crucial factors in reducing dependency tendencies.

References

4. *JAMA Internal Medicine*, "Prescription Opioid Use in the Management of Chronic Non-Cancer Pain," 2015.

5. *Pain Medicine Journal*, "Chronic Pain Management and the Risk of Opioid Dependency in Spinal Disorders," 2018.

6. CDC Report, *The Opioid Epidemic and Chronic Back Pain Solutions*, 2019.

7. *Journal of Neurosurgery*, "Assessing Opioid Dependency

<ol start="8">
<li>Annals of Internal Medicine, "Comparing Opioids with Non-Opioid Therapies for Back Pain Relief," 2019.</li>
<li>Complementary Therapies in Medicine, "Painkiller Reduction Linked to Chiropractic Care in Chronic Back Pain Patients," 2020.</li>
</ol>

Chronic back pain represents a dual crisis of physical discomfort and vulnerability to addiction. With emerging research strongly favoring non-invasive, long-term therapies, these alternatives not only prevent dependency but also provide sustainable pathways for spinal rehabilitation and overall well-being.

Closing Thoughts and References

This comprehensive documentation underscores how chiropractic care, spinal decompression, and GAG supplementation provide long-term, evidence-based alternatives to conventional disc treatments. The following sources provide further evidence supporting these findings:

References

1. Spine Journal, 2018

2. Journal of Pain Research, 2013

3. National Institutes of Health, GAIT, 2008

4. Journal of Manipulative and Physiological Therapeutics, 2021

5. Orthopaedic Research Journal, 2017

Through detailed research, this book has woven an intricate narrative of non-invasive approaches that prioritize patient health with scientifically validated outcomes, offering genuine hope for spinal recovery.

Emotional and Physical Impact

Studies have shown that unresolved post-surgical symptoms can lead to depression and chronic pain loops. Alternative therapies, however, address both physical pain and mental health consequences collaboratively.

Here are the references used for writing this chapter on the emotional impact of chronic pain and the role of counseling.

- American Psychological Association. (n.d.). Pain management. https://www.apa.org/topics/pain/management
- Cleveland Clinic. (n.d.). Chronic pain and mental health. https://my.clevelandclinic.org/health/articles/12051-chronic-pain-and-mental-health
- Dovepress. (n.d.). The link between chronic pain and depression: A biopsychosocial perspective. Journal of Pain Research. https://www.dovepress.com/the-link-between-chronic-pain-and-depression-a-biopsychosocial-perspec-peer-reviewed-fulltext-article-JPR
- GoodRx Health. (n.d.). Therapy for chronic pain: What works? https://www.goodrx.com/conditions/pain/therapy-for-chronic-pain
- Harvard Health Publishing. (n.d.). Chronic pain: The role of emotions. https://www.health.harvard.edu/mind-and-mood/chronic-pain-the-role-of-emotions
- Hospital for Special Surgery. (n.d.). The emotional impact of the pain experience. https://www.hss.edu/conditions_emotional-impact-pain-experience.asp
- Johns Hopkins Medicine. (n.d.). Chronic pain and emotional health. https://www.hopkinsmedicine.org/health/conditions-and-diseases/chronic-pain-and-emotional-health
- Mayo Clinic. (n.d.). Cognitive behavioral therapy

for chronic pain. https://www.mayoclinic.org/tests-procedures/cognitive-behavioral-therapy/about/pac-20384610

- National Institute of Mental Health. (n.d.). Chronic pain and depression. https://www.nimh.nih.gov/health/topics/chronic-pain-and-depression
- National Institute of Neurological Disorders and Stroke. (n.d.). Chronic pain information page. https://www.ninds.nih.gov/health-information/disorders/chronic-pain

Chapter 12
Take That First Step Towards Healing

Do you remember a time when your body felt completely free? When you could move without hesitation or discomfort, and the thought of pain never crossed your mind? That kind of ease and vitality is not just a distant memory—it's something you can reclaim. I want you to know that healing your spine, restoring your natural movement, and living the life you deserve is possible, and it starts with a decision. A decision you make today, right now.

Your spine is extraordinary. It's more than just a collection of bones—it's the very foundation of your body. Every twist, every bend, every breath—it's all supported by the silent work your spine does every single day. But like anything we rely on heavily, it needs care, attention, and the opportunity to heal when strain, injury, or degeneration occurs.

Maybe you've been living with back pain for years, or perhaps it's a new challenge that's suddenly disrupted your life. Whatever your situation, I'm here to tell you that you're not alone. And more importantly, there's hope. Real, tangible solutions exist—solutions that don't just mask the pain but address the root cause.

Reconnecting With Your Body

One of the things I've learned is that we often forget how connected we are to our bodies. We push through the discomfort, adjust our routines, or ignore the small signs that something might be wrong. But when your spine isn't functioning properly, it's not just your physical health that suffers—it affects your energy, your sleep, your productivity, and even your emotional well-being.

Chiropractic care is one of the most amazing tools for helping us reconnect with our bodies. Think of it as hitting a reset button, allowing your spine to find its proper alignment and giving your nervous system the space it needs to function correctly. Misaligned vertebrae—the ones causing discomfort, pinching nerves, and limiting your movements—can be gently guided back into their proper place. You don't just feel better physically; you feel lighter, like you're finally back in sync with yourself.

What I love most about chiropractic isn't just the relief it provides—though that's incredible—it's the empowerment. Every adjustment reminds you that your body is capable of healing. It shows you how remarkable and resilient your spine truly is when it's given the care it needs.

Releasing the Pressure

Now, I want you to picture something with me. Imagine your spine as a bridge, carrying the weight of your body every moment of the day. Over time, that weight—the constant pulling of gravity, poor posture, maybe an old injury—starts to take its toll. The bridge becomes compressed, tight, and strained. And the discs between your vertebrae—the soft cushions that should act as shock absorbers—begin to deteriorate under the pressure.

This is where spinal decompression therapy becomes a game-changer. Spinal decompression is like giving your spine the gift of space. It gently stretches and elongates the spine, easing the pressure on those discs and allowing them to "breathe" again.

Think of a sponge that's been dried out and flattened over time. When you give it water, it soaks it up, becoming plump and functional once more. That's exactly what decompression does for your spinal discs. It creates an environment where the discs can rehydrate, absorb nutrients, and start the healing process.

And the results? For so many people, it's freedom from pain that has followed them for years. It's the ability to sleep through the night without tossing and turning to find a comfortable position. It's being able to do things that once seemed out of reach—something as simple as picking up your kids or taking that long walk you've been avoiding.

The Hidden Heroes of Healing

But here's where the magic of healing truly comes together. Spinal decompression creates the space, while chiropractic care ensures alignment and balance. And then, there are glycosaminoglycans—those tiny, powerful molecules you've probably never thought about but are vital for your spinal health.

Glycosaminoglycans (or GAGs) are like the "hydration specialists" of your discs. They're what help your discs retain water, stay elastic, and do their job as the cushions between your vertebrae. When there's injury or degeneration, your discs lose these essential molecules. They become dried out, stiff, and far more prone to damage.

But the incredible thing is that GAG levels can be replenished. With the right nutrients, targeted therapies, and consistent care, your body can begin to rebuild these vital building blocks. It's a bit like planting seeds in a garden—at first, the changes aren't visible, but with time, nourishment, and effort, growth happens.

When GAGs are restored, your spinal discs regain their flexibility, their bounce, and their ability to support you without pain or resistance. This isn't just about avoiding more damage; it's about genuinely restoring what was lost.

Mental and Emotional Impact
of Chronic Pain

Chronic pain is more than just a physical condition—

it affects every part of a person's life, from emotional well-being to daily function. The frustration, anxiety, and isolation that often accompany long-term pain can create a cycle that's difficult to break. True healing requires addressing both the body and mind, which is why an integrative approach is essential. By combining advanced physical treatments like non-surgical spinal decompression with mental health support, patients can gain not only relief but also the tools to manage pain more effectively and reclaim their quality of life.

At Curis Functional Health, we believe in treating the whole person, not just the symptoms. Our approach blends cutting-edge technology with functional medicine and mental wellness strategies, ensuring that patients receive comprehensive, lasting care. Healing is a journey that requires both physical recovery and emotional resilience, and with the right support, relief is within reach. By embracing this holistic approach, patients can move beyond pain, regain control, and step into a future of strength, confidence, and renewed well-being.

A Journey Worth Starting

I know healing can feel overwhelming. It might seem like there are so many steps to take, so much time needed, and who knows if it will even work? But I also know this—nothing is more important than your health. Everything you want to do, everything you dream of experiencing, depends on your ability to move, to live free from pain, to feel at ease in your body.

And the good news is, you're not alone in this. Chiropractic care, spinal decompression, and strategies to replenish GAGs aren't just theories—they are real, proven approaches with the power to change lives. I've seen it happen. I've heard the stories of people who have felt trapped in their pain, only to find hope and healing through these methods.

All it takes is one step. One call, one appointment, one

decision to prioritize your healing.

Your Call to Action

If you're reading this, then you're already on the path to change. You've taken the time to learn about your spine and the tools available to heal it—that's an incredible first step. What comes next is up to you.

I'm asking you to take action. Start with a consultation, talk to a chiropractor, and learn about your spine's specific needs. Commit to making small changes in your daily life—pay attention to your posture, stretch, and move your body with care. Explore the therapies we've discussed and see how they fit into your own healing plan.

And most importantly, believe in your ability to heal. Your spine, your body—they want to recover. They want to function as they were meant to. And with the right support, they will.

This isn't just about pain relief—it's about reclaiming your freedom. It's about being able to play with your children, sit comfortably at your desk, dance at weddings, run marathons, or simply wake up without that nagging ache in your back.

Your spine is worth it. *You* are worth it.

Today, right now, choose to take that step. Reach out to a chiropractor. Learn about decompression therapy. Nourish your body in ways that support your spine. Because the sooner you start, the sooner you'll begin to feel what's possible.

You don't have to live with pain. You don't have to settle for limitations. Your spine has carried you this far—now it's your turn to care for it and allow it to heal.

The path to recovery is waiting. Take that first step and follow it. Your body, your mind, and your future self will thank you for it.

Chapter 13
Connecting with Dr. Stephanie Maj, Clinical Director of Curis Functional Health-Chicago Lakeview

Building a great relationship with your healthcare provider is key to feeling your best. Dr. Stephanie Maj, Clinical Director at Curis Functional Health-Chicago Lakeview, is here to provide caring, personalized support for better spinal health and overall wellness. Want to reach out to Dr. Maj and her team? It's easy—just head to gocuris.com/chicago-lakeview.

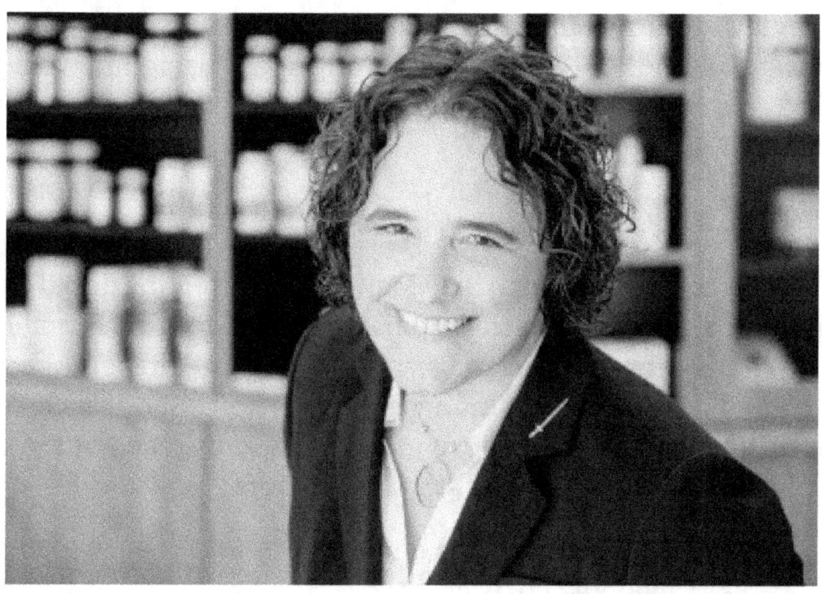

Email

The easiest way to get in touch with Dr. Maj is by shooting an email to drmaj@drmaj.com. Whether you've got questions, concerns, or need to book an appointment, just include your name, a quick note about what you need, and the best way to reach you. Dr. Maj and her team will reply quickly, so you'll get the help you need in no time!

Phone

Need help right away? Just give us a call at 773-528-8485! The friendly team at Curis Functional Health-Chicago Lakeview is here during office hours to answer your questions and get you set up with an appointment. Calling after hours? No problem—leave us a voicemail with your name, number, and what you need, and we'll get back to you ASAP!

Location and Office Hours

Dr. Maj is here to help at the Curis Functional Health-Chicago Lakeview clinic! You'll find us at 1442 W. Belmont Ave, Suite 1E, Chicago, IL 60657—a cozy, welcoming space designed with you in mind. We've got flexible hours to fit your busy schedule, so stop by and let's take care of you!

Social Media

Stay connected with Dr. Maj and Curis Functional Health-Chicago Lakeview on social media! We share tips on spinal health, pain management resources, and clinic updates to keep you informed and inspired. Got a quick question? Shoot us a DM! For anything more specific or private, it's better to reach out via email or phone. Follow along and stay in the loop!

- Instagram: @curis.chicago
- Facebook: curis.chicago
- Tik Tok: @curis.chicago

Take the First Step Toward Better Health

If you've been dealing with chronic pain, new symptoms,

or just want to focus on preventive care, reaching out to Dr. Stephanie Maj at Curis Functional Health-Chicago Lakeview could be a game-changer. Dr. Maj and her team are here to support you every step of the way with a compassionate, personalized approach that makes you feel truly cared for.

Why wait to take control of your health? Whether you prefer email, a quick call, or using their online booking system, that first step can make all the difference. Dr. Maj and her team are ready to help you find relief and start healing. They're excited to be part of your journey to a healthier, pain-free life. Your wellness matters—go ahead and reach out today!